Effective and Emerging Treatments in Pediatric Psychology

II0642964

Effective and Emerging Treatments in Pediatric Psychology

Anthony Spirito
Anne E. Kazak

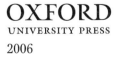

OXFORD
UNIVERSITY PRESS
2006

OXFORD
UNIVERSITY PRESS

Oxford University Press, Inc., publishes works that further
Oxford University's objective of excellence
in research, scholarship, and education.

Oxford   New York
Auckland   Cape Town   Dar es Salaam   Hong Kong   Karachi
Kuala Lumpur   Madrid   Melbourne   Mexico City   Nairobi
New Delhi   Shanghai   Taipei   Toronto

With offices in
Argentina   Austria   Brazil   Chile   Czech Republic   France   Greece
Guatemala   Hungary   Italy   Japan   Poland   Portugal   Singapore
South Korea   Switzerland   Thailand   Turkey   Ukraine   Vietnam

Published by Oxford University Press, Inc.
198 Madison Avenue, New York, New York 10016

www.oup.com

Oxford is a registered trademark of Oxford University Press

Library of Congress Cataloging-in-Publication Data
Spirito, Anthony.
Effective and emerging treatments in pediatric psychology / Anthony Spirito,
Anne E. Kazak.
p.   cm.
Includes bibliographical references and index.
ISBN-13: 978-0-19-515615-7; 978-0-19-518839-4 (pbk.)
ISBN 0-19-515615-3; 0-19-518839-X (pbk.)
1. Pediatrics—Psychological aspects. 2. Children—Diseases—Treatment—Psychological
aspects.   I. Kazak, Anne E.   II. Title.
RJ47.3.S65   2005
618.92—dc22   2005003884

9 8 7 6 5 4 3 2 1
Printed in the United States of America
on acid-free paper

To the children and families we serve

To our children, Emilia B. and Evan B. Spirito and Samuel C. Kazak

Contents

Introduction and Overview

Helping children with pediatric health problems and their families address psychological difficulties associated with their illnesses and treatments is essential in improving the quality of care children and families receive and in addressing the morbidity associated with pediatric illnesses. The field of pediatric psychology has been devoted, in large part, to developing and delivering interventions across a broad range of conditions and patient groups. These interventions are based on solid theories and reflect considerable progress over the past several decades in the translation of research into practice.

The treatment research literature in pediatric psychology is small but growing. An Empirically Supported Treatments Series was published in the *Journal of Pediatric Psychology* (*JPP*) from 1999 to 2001. Papers in this series helped to define the state of the art of pediatric psychology interventions at that time. In the interim, additional studies have been published, although the dissemination of treatments remains somewhat problematic. This book is designed to provide practicing clinicians and researchers with an update on treatments found to be effective in pediatric psychology as well as those that are emerging in the field and have promise of being proven effective as additional research is conducted.

A primary aim of this book is to provide sufficient detail regarding the interventions so that clinicians can implement in their practice those treatments shown to be empirically supported. At the same time, we provide details of clinical techniques in order to assist clinical researchers in developing research protocols that can be tested in future studies. An essential component of dissemination is access to intervention protocols. This book provides readers with access to treatment protocols developed by leading pediatric psychology researchers for the companion Web site for the book: www.oup.com/us/pediatricpsych. We believe this link will facilitate dissemination as readers may use these manuals in clinical work or contact the manual developers if interested in using or adapting the manuals for research protocols.

Besides access to manuals on the Web site, this book contains additional clinical material in its five parts. In the first part of this book, two chapters discuss the recent efforts in our field to document empirically supported and effective treatments and the role of treatment manuals in disseminating these effective treatments. In chapter 1, the roots of the empirically supported treatments "movement" are briefly reviewed as well as the outcomes of this effort specific to the field of pediatric psychology. Challenges associated with this approach to summarizing the treatment literature are also reviewed. The dissemination of clinical techniques through chapters in the book and the book's Web site are also described. Providing easy access to treatment manuals is the primary means by which this dissemination will occur. Consequently, chapter 2 reviews the pros and cons of using manualized treatments in clinical practice. Major controversies regarding the use of manuals, such as their effect on clinical judgment, difficulties in implementation when used with patients with comorbid conditions, and the effect of manualized treatments on therapeutic alliance, are reviewed. In this chapter we hope to allay undue concern regarding the use of manuals and encourage clinicians to experiment with their use in practice.

In the second part of this book, we provide two chapters that review details on individual and multiperson interventions. There is an emphasis on behavioral and cognitive behavioral protocols because they have been the most widely tested individual therapy approaches used in effective treatments in our field. Chapter 3, therefore, provides details on both behavioral and cognitive techniques that should be useful for clinicians. A detailed relaxation protocol is described, as is a problem-solving procedure. Cognitive-behavioral protocols for anger and anxiety control are also outlined. In chapter 4, the rationale and importance of a family/systems focus in pediatric psychology are reviewed as well as studies that support the efficacy of family, group, and other systemic interventions in pediatric psychology. An example of a manualized family intervention that has been empirically tested, the Surviving Cancer Competently Intervention Program (SCCIP), is described in detail.

In part III, two chapters examine problems that cut across medical conditions: pain and adherence to medical regimens. Chapter 5 on pain updates the literature on four types of pediatric pain: headaches, recurrent abdominal pain (RAP), procedure-related pain, and disease-related pain. The treatment literature on headaches and RAP has not advanced greatly since reviews were published in the *JPP* series several years ago. Nonetheless, behavioral treatment packages for these problems are sufficiently well developed that they may be employed in everyday clinical work. The use of biofeedback in the treatment of pediatric headaches is described in some detail to assist clinicians in the use of this procedure in practice. Behavioral treatments for procedure-related pain continue to be widely researched and have been shown to be effective across a wide age range as well as across different medical procedures. Dr. Lindsey Cohen of Georgia State University contributed guidelines for the use of distraction in preschoolers and a coping skills protocol for school-age children; Dr. Jessica Guite of The Children's Hospital of Philadelphia also provided helpful comments and contributions to chapter 5. Disease-related pain remains rather underinvestigated, and further work is clearly necessary in this area. We note some of the differences in cognitive-behavioral therapy protocols when employed for disease-related problems rather than other types of pain.

Regarding adherence to medical regimens, we review in chapter 6 the limited literature on recent treatment trials to improve regimen adherence. Only four such studies were identified, one for juvenile rheumatoid arthritis and three for asthma. Another trial to improve adherence to the cystic fibrosis (CF) regimen is discussed in chapter 10. These additional studies have not resulted in any one treatment approach being considered well established. Nonetheless, the behavioral approaches currently used to address adherence problems are outlined in the hopes that future studies to improve adherence will be devised and tested. Challenges to conducting research on adherence to medical regimens, such as measurement issues, are significant. Also reviewed are factors that affect implementation, such as the role of beliefs and culture on patient acceptance of intervention strategies.

In part IV, chapters 7 through 9, we review the literature on three common childhood problems: nocturnal enuresis, encopresis, and sleep problems. In each of these chapters we update the intervention literature first and then describe clinical procedures for the different problems. For childhood encopresis, we review both medical management and behavioral approaches to toileting. Drs. Lisa Opipari-Arrigan of the University of Michigan and Michael Mellon of the Mayo Clinic provided very useful input into these management strategies. In chapter 7 on nocturnal enuresis, we note that the urine alarm is a well-established intervention and that no further research is necessary to demonstrate its effectiveness. We provide clinical guidelines on the use of urine alarms and also describe two newer approaches to managing nighttime wettings: waking children when their bladder is filled before they wet the bed, and using a miniature bladder volume measurement instrument that signals an alarm when the bladder reaches a specified volume. In chapter 9 on sleep problems, we review studies on extinction and graduated extinction and provide clinical guidelines for the use of these procedures. Two alternative approaches to managing early childhood sleep problems—scheduled awakenings and positive routines—are also reviewed. Individual and family factors that affect treatment acceptability and, in turn, treatment implementation are also discussed. Dr. Holly Sindelar of Brown University provided useful guidance on strategies used to manage childhood sleep problems, along with a review and other helpful comments regarding this chapter.

In the final part of the book, we review emerging treatments for children with CF. CF was chosen for inclusion because of the critical importance of adhering to the CF medical regimen in order for the disease to be properly managed. In addition, we chose CF to review because two senior investigators in the field, Drs. Alexandra Quittner of the University of Miami and Lori Stark, have provided readers access to the treatment manuals they have been testing to improve adherence to medical regimens for children with CF. Neither of these treatment protocols has been tested by other researchers, but both show promise as being effective. Dr. Stark, of the Cincinnati Children's Hospital Medical Center, also provided a review and helpful comments regarding this chapter.

This book was designed to be useful to both clinicians and clinical researchers alike. Details regarding clinical techniques used in a number of studies have been included to assist clinicians. The inclusion of manuals on this book's Web site should encourage researchers to develop and test protocols with new samples of children. We hope that these two approaches will result in advancing the field and improving the quality of care provided to children, adolescents, and families.

We wish to acknowledge the many pediatric psychologists whose research and clinical contributions have made possible the work we describe in this book. We also wish to give special thanks to our colleagues at Brown University (A.S.) and The Children's Hospital of Philadelphia (A.E.K.). We are fortunate to work with teams of exceptionally collegial, clinically wise, and research-savvy individuals. Special thanks are extended to the 20 classes of Brown University pediatric psychology interns and postdoctoral fellows for their contributions to this work and to the SCCIP research teams in Philadelphia for their dedication to developing effective and clinical meaningful interventions for cancer survivors and their families. We also thank Kathleen Bennett for patiently preparing and revising numerous drafts of the manuscript.

TREATMENT RESEARCH
AND PRACTICE

1 Effective Treatments in Pediatric Psychology

Psychologists working in pediatric settings are action-oriented health care professionals charged with translating psychological research into clinical practice. Pediatric psychologists function in a variety of roles, but in nearly all positions, effective treatments for ameliorating difficult cognitive, behavioral, emotional, and family concerns are essential components of practice. In addition, the expectation is for the delivery of prompt and effective treatments, within a collaborative multidisciplinary framework.

Pediatric psychologists have been quite successful in delivering effective treatments, particularly when the treatments are based on well-established behavioral and cognitive-behavioral approaches. As scientist-practitioners, pediatric psychologists are also dedicated to the development of the scientific literature. This area of work has been successful, too, with a large body of research providing background on important characteristics of various pediatric psychology populations.

This background research provides the foundation for treatment research. However, the percentage of research dedicated to evaluating the outcomes of intervention approaches is small. For example, the current and three previous editors of the *Journal of Pediatric Psychology* (*JPP*), the major outlet for research in pediatric psychology, have noted the small number of intervention studies submitted and published (R. Brown, 2003; Kazak, 2002b; La Greca, 1997; Roberts, 1992). Although there is some indication that more intervention papers have been published during recent years than previously, research in pediatric psychology has emphasized assessment and explicative research rather than intervention. However, research on intervention effectiveness is critical, particularly in light of our national focus on health care costs and related emphasis on treatment guidelines. The lack of research on treatment outcomes is a major concern facing our field. It is our hope that this book, and its associated Web site,

3

described below, will both spark ideas for intervention research *and* provide a means for it to be conducted with greater success and fewer barriers.

Evidence-Based Practice in Pediatric Psychology

In this chapter we review the relevant background on empirically supported treatments in pediatric psychology and summarize the findings of a series of 11 treatment review papers published in *JPP* between 1999 and 2001. We extract the major achievements and their implications for practice while also highlighting areas of challenge and needs for further development in order to further promote the science and practice of pediatric psychology.

Each of the 11 review papers focused on a specific topic. Four were related to different aspects of pediatric pain—headache (Holden, Deichmann, & Levy, 1999), recurrent abdominal pain (Janicke & Finney, 1999), procedure-related pain (Powers, 1999), and disease-related pain (Walco, Sterling, Conte, & Engel, 1999). Two papers focused on topics related to eating: severe feeding problems (Kerwin, 1999) and obesity (Jelalian & Saelens, 1999). Three papers addressed the common childhood behavioral concerns of enuresis (Mellon & McGrath, 2000), encopresis and constipation (M. McGrath, Mellon, & Murphy, 2000), and bedtime refusal and night wakening (Mindell, 1999). Two papers were devoted to major areas of pediatric psychology practice: disease-related symptoms (McQuaid & Nassau, 1999) and adherence to medical treatments (Lemanek, Kamps, & Chung, 2001).

The idea for these papers was developed in collaboration with a committee of the Society of Pediatric Psychology (SPP). This committee emerged from the broader initiatives on empirically supported treatments of Division 12 (Society of Clinical Psychology) of the American Psychological Association. The articles used criteria established by a subcommittee of the Task Force on Effective Psychosocial Interventions, based within Division 12. The criteria were altered slightly for pediatric psychology interventions, due to considerations such as the low incidence of pediatric illnesses and the resulting difficulties with small sample sizes (Spirito, 1999).

In order to be considered a *well-established* intervention, it was necessary that there be two good between-group experiments that demonstrate efficacy in one of two ways: (a) showing superiority to a pill, psychological placebo, or alternative treatment or (b) demonstrating equivalence to an already established treatment in studies with adequate statistical power. Another way in which an intervention could be deemed well established was if there was a series of nine or more well-designed single-case experiments that included comparison to another treatment. Finally, two multiple baseline designs by independent investigators were also accepted. The studies also needed to describe the samples thoroughly, and outcomes must have been reported by two independent investigators. In the category of *probably efficacious,* two studies showing that the treatment was more effective than a wait-list control were required, or otherwise meeting somewhat relaxed criteria from the well-established interventions (e.g., it was not necessary to have been replicated by two independent groups). A treatment protocol was required, although not a manual. *Promising* interventions were those for which there were positive outcomes for one well-controlled study or a small series of single-case studies, or two or more well-controlled studies by the same investigator.

The articles in this series cover a broad literature and yet present data based on strict criteria and with focused questions. Table 1.1 summarizes the conclusions of the papers in the series. Four general themes, described below, can be extracted.

- *The size of the literature is small but sufficient. The number of papers published per area ranged from 9 to 42.* The median number of papers reviewed was 30. Although the quality of the studies varies and some of the reviews with a smaller set of papers make generalizability more difficult, 30 studies on a topic appear to be a reasonable size on which to draw conclusions. In addition, one of the areas with a smaller number of studies (procedure-related pain) shows a very strong congruence across studies. Thus, readers can feel confidence in basing treatment decisions on a number of these literature reviews.
- *Behavioral and cognitive-behavioral approaches dominate.* The treatments are heavily focused on behavioral and cognitive-behavioral approaches. This is not surprising, given the roots of pediatric psychology in clinical and child clinical psychology. Clearly, behavioral interventions lend themselves to empirical research and show efficacy across a range of pediatric problems. They are an important component of our treatment regimens and can be recommended across many situations. However, it is essential that other treatment modalities continue to be developed and evaluated and that innovation in intervention continues to be valued in our field.
- *"Probably efficacious" and promising interventions are widely available.* All but one of the reviews provide recommendations for one or more efficacious or probably efficacious interventions in their respective areas. Overall, 11 interventions were judged to be efficacious for seven

Table 1.1. Summary of *Journal of Pediatric Psychology* Empirically Supported Treatments Series Reviews

Topic	Studies (N)	Well-established/efficacious	Probably efficacious	Promising
Headache	31	Relaxation/self-hypnosis	Biofeedback	Combining approaches
Recurrent abdominal pain	9		Cognitive-behavioral therapy	Fiber
Procedure-related pain	13	Cognitive-behavioral therapy		
Disease-related pain	12			Cognitive-behavioral therapy
Severe feeding disorders	29	Differential attention Positive reinforcement + manual guidance		Extinction Swallowing induction
Obesity	42	Multicomponent behavioral intervention (children)		Multicomponent behavioral intervention (adolescents)
Nocturnal enuresis	39	Urine alarm	Full-Spectrum Home Training	Hypnosis
Encopresis and constipation	42	Urine alarm + "Dry Bed"	Positive reinforcement (with and without fiber) Biofeedback + medical intervention	
Bedtime refusal and night wakings	41	Extinction Parent education	Gradual extinction Scheduled awakenings	Positive routines
Disease-related symptoms	30	Electromyographic biofeedback (asthma) Imagery (chemotherapy)	Relaxation (asthma) Distraction + relaxation (chemotherapy)	Family therapy (asthma) Video games (chemotherapy)
Regimen adherence	23		Organizational strategies Behavioral strategies Multicomponent packages	Educational Behavioral Cognitive-behavioral therapy

presenting problems. An additional six interventions were judged to be probably efficacious in four areas where efficacious interventions were described (headache, nocturnal enuresis, bedtime refusal/night wakings, and disease-related symptoms). Six other interventions were judged to be probably efficacious in three areas that did not have any well-established (efficacious) interventions: recurrent abdominal pain, encopresis, and regimen adherence. Perhaps the largest collective disappointment in the reviews is the lack of support for interventions at the highest tier of the empirically supported treatment categories: well established/efficacious. However, the criteria for these categories are rigorous and are cause for reflection and redirection in future work. There were many interesting and probably important studies that were not sufficiently rigorous to be included as supporting evidence.

- *Integrative interventions are promising.* Several of the treatments noted to be effective as well as several in the promising category include interventions that incorporate more than one treatment approach. In some cases, this may be the combination of two behavioral or cognitive-behavioral techniques (e.g., relaxation plus distraction). In other cases, the multidisciplinary focus of pediatric health care is obvious, with medical treatments (e.g., fiber, sedation, medication) combined with psychological intervention approaches showing efficacy. Other treatment modalities may include several different psychological therapies (e.g., individual behaviorally oriented approaches for children combined with family treatment). In each case, these integrative approaches may prove to be more effective and more responsive to the needs of children, families, and medical staff than exclusive reliance on one treatment approach.

Challenges Associated With Effective Interventions in Pediatric Psychology

The goals of this book include providing readers with an informed critique of intervention research across a variety of areas of practice within pediatric psychology so that they can more readily access effective treatments and participate in the ongoing evaluation of treatment protocols. As such, it is important to reflect on the current state of the related research and to consider the challenges that we face in delivering and evaluating interventions.

Controversies Surrounding Empirically Supported Treatments

There are many controversies surrounding the definition and evolution of empirically supported treatments, evidence-based practice, and practice guidelines. It
is unlikely, and probably undesirable, to think that we will evolve a set of treatment parameters that are indisputably effective and immune to challenge by the
development of novel intervention approaches. The criteria used in the *JPP* review
papers and those discussed throughout this book do not imply unconditional
endorsement of the *JPP* Empirically Supported Treatments Series criteria or of
any other particular criteria for determining treatment efficacy. Our interest is in
promoting rigorous and clinically meaningful research. The existing treatment
evaluation criteria are reasonable starting points.

Critiques Specific to the JPP Series

Drotar (2002) raises three important criticisms of the *JPP* series. First, the vast
majority of intervention studies reviewed do not include effect sizes. By emphasizing statistical significance (usually in a between-groups or pre-post design),
larger samples are likely to yield statistically significant findings but may mask
clinically important findings. As Drotar (2002) points out, inclusion of effect
size data would facilitate comparisons across studies.

Second, Drotar (2002) notes that the reviews do not provide sufficient
emphasis on the clinical significance of the findings. This is critically important
and can be at least partially addressed at the design level of interventions to show
changes and effects that may not be detectable using standard statistical analyses of change, for example, showing how individuals have changed from their
baseline scores after intervention, using diagnostic criteria to show improvement, and assessing subjective evaluations of intervention acceptability and
importance as well as the impact of the intervention on others besides the child
(e.g., family members, teachers, peers, staff). A related point concerns the general absence of psychopathology in children with pediatric health care problems
and their parents (Kazak, Rourke, & Crump, 2003). Most children with chronic
illness, for example, are psychologically healthy and capable of adaptive coping,
as are their families. The types of changes that may occur over time may not be
detected using instruments designed to document psychopathology.

Drotar's (2002) third point laments the disconnection between theory and
intervention in many of the studies reviewed. He correctly points out that when
studies drift from a clear conceptual framework, it becomes more difficult (if

not impossible) to identify the mechanisms of change and to sustain a program of research that advances and improves outcomes.

Diversity in Pediatric Psychology Interventions and Generalizability

Another important concern related to intervention outcome studies in pediatric psychology is the lack of attention to issues related to ethnic and socioeconomic factors (Clay, Mordhorst, & Lehn, 2002). These authors tallied information on whether 71 papers included in the *JPP* Empirically Supported Treatments Series review papers on asthma, cancer, diabetes, and obesity reported race/ethnicity or socioeconomic status (SES) and also examined whether these articles discussed possible moderating effects of cultural variables. The results are striking: 27% of the papers reviewed reported race, and 18% reported SES. A small subset (6%) addressed moderating effects of culture. Similarly, Kazak (2005) notes the consistent and striking sampling in interventions related to children with cancer and their families. In cancer and other illness groups, samples are overwhelmingly Caucasian and also tend to rely on child or maternal report without representation of fathers and other family members.

Comprehensiveness of Topics

The breadth of intervention activities of pediatric psychologists is not fully represented in this series of papers. From the series, one would have the impression that pediatric psychologists intervene primarily with individual children to reduce pain (chronic and acute), to resolve behavioral problems related to elimination and sleep, to reduce symptoms associated with treatment, and to improve adherence to medical treatments. While it would be difficult to argue with this picture of hospital-based pediatric psychology intervention, it is not a complete picture. Pediatric psychologists, for example, are involved in preventive intervention research, have partnerships in collaborative studies with multidisciplinary colleagues, conduct research with families and in schools, and develop and test interventions that promote well-being and positive adaptation as well as decreasing specific symptoms.

Research Models, Modalities, and Activities

The research accomplishments of pediatric psychologists have solidified our reputation as scientists. However, some of our research activities may need to shift in order to continue to provide rigorous, meaningful, and creative intervention research in the future. It is, for example, very difficult to accrue sufficient sample sizes for randomized clinical trials at one site, particularly if the disease, treatment, or developmental stage should be defined narrowly. Similarly, the goal of including ethnically diverse samples of sufficient size will generally necessitate data collection at multiple sites. Multisite studies are, of course, not a panacea and have their own inherent difficulties. However, by identifying eligible participants at multiple institutions, the possibilities for increasing rigor and generalizability increase.

Another difficulty inherent in pediatric psychology intervention research relates to the developmental stage of much of the work. A first trial, for example, of a psychological intervention for a specific pediatric patient group might take several years to complete, particularly if the participants must fit specific eligibility criteria. At the end of the trial, replication is often not an appropriate option. That is, rather than repeat the original intervention, study results may point to the need for refinement in the protocol. Given this reality, we are unlikely to replicate studies and thereby will have difficulty meeting criteria for empirically supported treatments.

Promoting the Use of Effective Interventions: Overview of This Book

In preparing this book, a primary goal was to reduce barriers to the use of effective treatment approaches by pediatric psychologists. In order to do so, we explored means by which treatment manuals and related data on the outcomes of interventions could be disseminated more readily to practicing pediatric psychologists. We also wished to improve access to investigators doing research on interventions who might be interested in collaborating by conducting related studies at their sites. In sum, we tried to facilitate the use of effective interventions and to also help grow the database of information necessary for the ongoing development of this work.

This book attempts to accomplish the goals described above in three ways. First, we include chapters on individual and multiperson approaches to treatment. These chapters contain descriptions of different treatment protocols as well as specific scripts for certain procedures, for example, relaxation and problem solving. These materials, we hope, will be useful to both clinicians in their day-to-day practice and clinical researchers in implementing and developing research protocols. Second, in the chapters on specific problems, such as enuresis, clinical research protocols are described at some length, and "helpful hints" about the use of these protocols in clinical practice are described. And third, an essential part of this book is its companion Web site (www.oup.com/us/pediatricpsych). In preparing this book, we have been fortunate to have leading pediatric psychology intervention researchers (Drs. Alexandra Quittner and Lori Stark) generously provide treatment manuals for their interventions, which are accessible online. Their complete manuals for the treatment of specific problems encountered in the treatment of children with cystic fibrosis (feeding difficulties and adherence to the treatment regimen) are provided on the Web site. Our intent was twofold: to provide easy access to intervention protocols that are being empirically tested and also to make available up-to-date information (from the authors of the protocols), including new and emerging findings from their research laboratories. We will provide easy access to intervention protocols by updating this Web site annually with additional treatment manuals for problems encountered in the practice of pediatric psychology. This procedure will be a joint effort of the authors of this volume and the SPP. It is our intention to add new manuals and provide updated information on the studies supporting the different clinical research protocols as well as provide input on how to best use these protocols in clinical practice. Initially, the Web site will be very basic and will primarily function as a convenient site to download manuals.

Use of the manuals includes an agreement to use the protocol as written, to communicate with the author regarding standard information about their use, and to agree to share data with the principal investigator from any studies conducted with the protocol.

The authors and the SPP believe this approach to making treatment manuals widely available to pediatric psychologists will provide much-needed impetus to advancing treatment research in our field. In addition, it will provide easy access to emerging and effective treatment protocols for practicing clinicians, which will in turn lead to improved quality care for pediatric patients.

2 Treatment Manuals and Clinical Practice

Translating psychotherapy research findings from the laboratory to the clinic is a challenge but is necessary in order to facilitate the partnership between research and practice. One practical obstacle clinicians encounter is simply obtaining the treatment manuals used in research trials (Weisz, Donenberg, Han, & Weiss, 1995). Providing access to treatment manuals is the primary means by which this book and its companion Web site aim to achieve the goal of disseminating promising and effective treatments. Treatment manuals owe their popularity to their use in controlled psychotherapy research protocols, such as the National Institute of Mental Health's Collaborative Study of Depression. Now considered mandatory in psychotherapy research, manuals have begun to find their way into clinical practice. The recent promotion of empirically supported treatments has accelerated the dissemination of treatment manuals to clinicians. Manuals are purported to be the most efficient means of disseminating treatment approaches to providers and trainees, especially those who may have limited formal training in a specific procedure. Manualized treatments are rapidly becoming the cornerstone for implementing clinical practice or "best practices" guidelines (Strosahl, 1998). Nonetheless, the use of manuals for treatment in clinical practice is not without controversy. In this chapter, pros and cons regarding the use of manuals in clinical practice are described.

There are a number of advantages to manualized treatments. Manuals are considered useful by many clinicians because they provide explicit guidelines for conducting treatment as well as details about treatment techniques. The structure of manuals may promote transportability to clinical settings (Kazdin, Kratochwill, & VandenBos, 1986) and reduce the probability of idiosyncratic decision making (Wilson, 1997). Thus, manuals may also enable providers to deliver treatments with at least a modicum of treatment fidelity (Strosahl, 1998). This structure also benefits clinicians with varying levels of experience by focusing treatment on specific problems and goals (Chambless, 1996). Finally, the structure of manuals, which includes specifying the goals and techniques of therapy and providing feedback regarding progress, may also facilitate patient involvement in the therapy (Wilson, 1998).

Introducing treatment manuals into everyday practice is considered problematic by some. Some question the feasibility of employing manual-based treatment protocols in a typical clinical practice. Specifically, most clinical research protocols are intensive, whereas most care in clinical practices is based on cost efficiency. Most clinics do not place an incentive on completion of thorough treatment protocols when waiting lists are long. Because most manuals were originally designed for psychotherapy research protocols, they may not always be user friendly, which in turn affects their acceptability by clinicians. Some clinicians question whether the advent of manualized treatment may make it necessary to learn and use multiple manuals for the variety of presenting problems encountered in clinical practice. Other clinicians express concern that manualized treatments may not be acceptable to some patients (Addis, Wade, & Hatgis, 1999). The most prominent concerns about the use of manuals in practice include the effects of manuals on clinical judgment, the flexibility of manuals in accounting for individual differences, the use of manuals for complex and comorbid conditions, the effects of manual-based protocols on the therapeutic alliance, and the potential negative effects of manuals on developing new treatments.

Clinical Judgment and Manualized Treatment

Because therapists are typically trained to develop individualized case formulations and treatment plans, it is not surprising that clinicians object to the potential negative effects of manuals on clinical judgment. Two major constraints on clinical judgment are described: lack of attention to individual differences and too great an adherence to a theoretical model.

Many clinicians question whether individual differences, such as cognitive level, family context, the patient's belief system and expectations regarding therapy, and cultural factors (Kaslow et al., 1997), are adequately addressed in manualized treatments. And in the treatment of children, developmental factors must also be considered (Weisz, 1998), which makes the use of manuals even more challenging. Proponents of manuals argue that these factors are important but can be addressed in most manualized treatments. In addition, although individualizing treatment to the specific problem behaviors of the child or adolescent is important, the data supporting the matching of treatments to clients are not very strong (Project MATCH; Longabaugh & Wirtz, 2001; Nelson-Gray, Herbert, Sigmon, & Brannon, 1989). Thus, treatment outcome may be less dependent on individualized treatment than most clinicians might predict. Ultimately, the degree of applicability of a manual-based treatment to an individual child will depend on whether the manual is designed to address causal factors that are pertinent to the child's problems (S. Haynes, Kaholokula, & Nelson, 1999).

Treatment manuals are typically based on one theoretical model, whereas in clinical practice it is common for clinicians to integrate therapy techniques from different theoretical models. Thus, clinicians raise concern about potential negative effects of manuals on therapist case conceptualization. Researchers assert that manuals are most effective when they are "driven by the framework, not by the specific techniques" (Kendall, Chu, Gifford, Hayes, & Nauta, 1998, p. 179). In such manuals, theoretical models provide overarching goals for treatment and specific goals for each session, while the procedures in the manual guide the therapist toward achieving these goals (Kendall et al., 1998). Thus, the degree of success of any treatment program will depend at least in part on how well clinicians understand the model being used in the treatment manual.

Flexibility and Use of the Manuals

The invariant sequence of treatment components in some manualized treatments has been criticized as interfering with therapy. More and more frequently, however, treatment manuals have increased the flexibility with which their components are delivered. In the most flexible of manual-based treatments, those based on treatment principles rather than techniques (e.g., Persons, 1991), these concerns are not very significant. Most other types of manuals now present a number of different techniques from which only a few are chosen as core techniques to be implemented across patients. Other techniques may be chosen based on both patient presentation and patient progress. In addition, in many protocols, therapists can delay, eliminate, or speed up the use of certain techniques in the outlined sequence of treatment. Psychotherapy researchers have also begun to write about ways to make manuals flexible and creative for children (Kendall et al., 1998).

Even the most flexible manuals need to have decision rules so that the treatment applied to patients with similar difficulties is comparable (Henin, Otto, &

Reilly-Harrington, 2001). Modular approaches, that is, modules for specific problems and techniques, are particularly conducive to flexible treatments if decision rules can be applied as to what modules should be used for pinpointed problems (Eifert, Schulte, Zvolensky, Lejuez, & Lau, 1997). Finally, therapist-rated flexibility of a manual is not necessarily associated with a better outcome of therapy (e.g., Kendall & Chu, 2000). The more individual modifications are made in practice, the greater the likelihood that the treatment may not be as effective as that delivered in the original research study (Schulte & Eifert, 2002).

Another concern is that there may be some therapeutic strategies commonly used in practice that do not translate very well into manual form (Eifert, Evans, & McKendrick, 1990). In turn, this may increase resistance of clinicians to the use of manuals or limit the types of treatment that might be manualized. Manuals have also been criticized for not allowing therapists to adequately respond to important issues that might arise in sessions that are relevant to the patient's ultimate outcome but are not covered in the treatment manual (Kendall & Chu, 2000). However, most proponents of manualized treatments allow deviations from the protocol when events arise that interfere with the manual-based treatment protocol. The more manuals provide practical guidelines and discuss the common clinical problems that may occur, the more likely it is that manuals will be widely embraced by clinicians. Guidelines for engaging the patient in the process of treatment and overcoming resistance to treatment are particularly useful and can be found in some newer manuals.

Despite the concerns about flexibility, it should be noted that, in clinical practice, therapists often start with a particular treatment approach and continue with this approach, even if it is less than successful (Kendall, Kipnis, & Otto-Salaj, 1992). In addition, in the field of pediatric psychology, there are some specific treatment protocols for specific presenting problems, for example, feeding disorders or encopresis, in which a prescribed set and order of techniques are recommended. In such cases lack of flexibility does not typically pose implementation difficulties.

Complex Patients, Comorbidity, and Manuals

A major objection of clinicians to manuals revolves around the observation that patients typically present with multiple problems and comorbid diagnoses that may not be appropriate for a single treatment manual. Because most manuals have been developed for research projects, manualized treatments are typically devised for persons with a specific disorder or a presenting problem. However, patients with a common diagnosis or presenting problem are not necessarily alike. Persons (1991) notes that individuals with the same diagnosis may be experiencing very different problems. Similarly, many presenting problems cannot be neatly categorized. Structured manuals tend to ignore these functional aspects of behavior. These individual differences also suggest that not all persons with the same disorder require all components of a manualized protocol, and in fact, such an approach might lead to negative effects of treatment (Persons, 1991).

Strosahl (1998) notes that there is no reason to think most manualized treatments wouldn't work with less than diagnostically pure disorders. Indeed, manualized treatments have been found to be effective for clients that have comorbid conditions (Persons, Bostrom, & Bertagnolli, 1999). Although complex and multifaceted problem behaviors of an individual may be more likely to require individualized treatment approaches (Eifert et al., 1997), certain patterns of comorbidity may be more or less amenable to a single treatment approach. Manualized treatments targeting one problem or disorder may also lead to clinical improvements in comorbid conditions (Wilson, 1998). If improvement does not occur, treatment can be sequential (Wilson, 1998). Alternatively, therapy might be delivered concurrently in a protocol that integrates two manual-based treatments. In such cases, it may not be possible to fully treat the comorbid condition, and therapists will need to pick particular problems to target in the treatment. Another possibility for positive outcome occurs when presenting problems in different disorders are functionally related and therefore both may respond to the treatment of a symptom in the identified problem disorder.

The Therapeutic Alliance and Manual-Based Treatment

Clinicians also raise concerns about the effects of manuals on establishing the therapeutic relationship. Indeed, one study (Castonguay, Goldfried, Wiser, Rave, & Hayes, 1996) found that in a small sample of depressed adults being treated with cognitive therapy, increased adherence to the cognitive techniques in the manual negatively affected the therapeutic alliance. Such a finding is problematic because the therapeutic relationship is the most important means by which patients are encouraged to emit behaviors that facilitate treatment, such as self-disclosure and agreeing to cooperate and try out proposed interventions (Schulte & Eifert, 2002). Thus, the quality of treatment delivery is directly related to the therapeutic relationship. Some therapists do have trouble following manual guidelines while at the same time attending to the therapeutic relationship. However, this is usually the case early in the use of manuals when novice therapists are unfamiliar and anxious about using a manualized treatment, feel unprepared or unskilled in the therapy, and therefore may be more rigid in their application of the treatment tasks in the manual (Kendall, 1998). There may be a learning curve associated with standardized treatments in order to ensure that the therapeutic relationship is optimized while delivering the treatment.

Clinicians will need to balance several competing tasks to most effectively treat clients using a manual. Addis, Hatgis, Soysa, and Zaslavsky (1999) point out two questions pertinent to the therapeutic relationship that therapists must ask themselves as they deliver manualized treatments. First, "Am I too focused on the individual or too focused on adhering to the manual?" Responses to this question include: The treatment works for a range of people, so don't overindividualize; the manual provides a general framework; and focus on the aspects of this person's presentation that are particularly applicable to a treatment manual. And second, "Am I not sufficiently attending to the therapeutic relationship or am I too concerned with the therapeutic alliance at the expense of the manual components?" Responses to this question include: Decide on the type of therapeutic relationship that best facilitates treatment techniques; and explore how the manualized techniques can strengthen the therapeutic alliance.

If manual developers describe the components of the therapeutic alliance that are most pertinent to a particular manualized treatment, clients may be best served. Thus, manualized treatment does not necessarily mean that the therapeutic alliance is negatively affected. Indeed, in one study at a community mental health clinic, clients rated the therapeutic relationship superior in treatment delivered by therapists using manuals as compared with treatment delivered by therapists employing standard care (Addis, Wade, et al., 1999).

Emerging Treatment Approaches and Manuals

One last concern commonly mentioned by clinicians is the potential negative effects of manual-based treatments on emerging and innovative treatment techniques and protocols. That is, strict adherence to manualized and inflexible protocols might stifle the development of innovative treatment approaches. However, as we have tried to impress upon the reader in this chapter, flexible manuals that require skilled therapists who attend to the therapeutic relationship and nonspecific factors are rapidly becoming the standard in manual-based treatments. Flexible manuals require clinical judgment and the ability to choose appropriate treatment techniques for a given problem. These conditions are no less conducive to the development of new and innovative treatment techniques than is "usual care." In fact, when consistent difficulties arise in the course of implementing a manualized treatment, clinicians using these protocols will be forced to try innovative approaches. Successful innovations may be more likely to be disseminated broadly when there is a large group of clinicians using the same manualized protocol (Addis, Wade, et al., 1999).

Conclusions

Ultimately, the success of manuals in clinical practice will depend on how useful clinicians find these manualized protocols in their practice. Godley, White, Diamond, Passetti, and Titus (2001) surveyed therapist reactions to the use of manualized treatment protocols in a five-site field study for adolescents who abused marijuana. Therapists commented positively on the structure of the protocol ("It is very clear—very concrete," p. 410), ease of use, focus ("gives me a sense of where I need to go," p. 410), creativity ("there's more room than some people may think to individualize and personalize the therapy," p. 410), and flexibility ("it doesn't restrict you in the flexibility to meet an individual kid's or family's needs," p. 410). The most common criticism was the constraining effect a structured manual had on therapy style. Godley et al. (2001) were also able to elicit feedback from the therapists on deviations from the manual. These deviations occurred when serious clinical issues arose: logistics (e.g., patient arriving late and having a shortened session), uncooperativeness of the patients, inappropriateness of the material (e.g., the examples given in the manual were not realistic for a particular child), and when family issues needed to be addressed. Overall, however, it appears that manualized treatments were well received and well implemented by clinicians.

Although concerns about incorporating manual-based treatments into clinical practice are legitimate, many of the issues raised regarding manualized treatments pertain to all forms of psychotherapy. This chapter has outlined responses and solutions to these concerns that, when taken together, suggest that therapists can learn to appreciate the positive aspects of manuals.

The more clinicians use these manuals and provide feedback to their developers, the better these manuals will become and the more widespread their use will be.

II INTERVENTION APPROACHES

3 Individual Therapies

Individual treatment with children and adolescents is an important aspect of working in the field of pediatric psychology. Supportive psychotherapy is probably the most commonly employed therapeutic approach used with pediatric patients. This is particularly true when helping children with a chronic illness cope with the stress of their disease and its treatment. In the Empirically Supported Treatments Series in the *Journal of Pediatric Psychology* (*JPP*), however, 11 topic areas were reviewed, and all of the seven individual interventions rated as well established were behavioral or cognitive-behavioral procedures. This is not surprising given the fact that this is true of the general psychotherapy literature with children and adults. In addition, many of the problems encountered by pediatric psychologists naturally lend themselves to contingency management approaches (e.g., sleep onset difficulties, self-control, and pain management). Therefore, cognitive-behavioral approaches are described in this chapter. Relaxation is the most common behavioral procedure used in a variety of protocols. Consequently, relaxation is described in detail in this chapter. Cognitive techniques are typically used in self-management protocols. Problem-solving and cognitive coping strategies are most common and are reviewed below. Finally, affect management protocols have occasionally been referred to in the *JPP* Empirically Supported Treatments Series studies and are also discussed in this chapter.

Behavioral Techniques: Relaxation Training

Relaxation training is often incorporated into behavioral protocols for pediatric patients, often to help control pain and/or anxiety. The goal of relaxation training is to induce a physiologic state that is incompatible with negative emotional or physical sensations. Although there are numerous descriptions of relaxation training, most are geared toward adults. There are special considerations and adaptations that may be necessary when working with pediatric populations. These are detailed below.

Tailoring the relaxation procedure to the child will enhance its effectiveness and depends on such factors as the child's age and developmental level, presenting problem, temperament, visual imaging skills, and medical presentation. One of the first decisions to be made is the type of relaxation to be taught: imagery, autogenic training, diaphragmatic breathing, or meditative breathing. *Imagery-based relaxation* procedures are a relatively passive means of producing relaxation that takes advantage of visualization abilities often heightened in childhood. In such procedures, the child is asked to visualize a favored activity or pleasant scene. By focusing on such a visual image, concentration is enhanced and relaxation results. Pleasant scenes or activities can vary widely and will often not be consistent with an adult's pleasant image. For example, whereas many adults consider lying on a beach a relaxing activity, most children find this boring and would prefer other beach images, such as swimming underwater, building a sand castle, and so forth. Sports imagery may be useful with some children, such as imagining a basketball player who calms down at the foul line before attempting to shoot under pressure (Sommers-Flanagan & Sommers-Flanagan, 1995).

Although clinicians typically use an image a child chooses, there are situations in which certain visual images may be contraindicated. For example, for a child who anticipates being hospitalized for an extended period of time, such as over the summer, a beach scene might induce relaxation but also lead to feelings of sadness after the relaxation procedure ends because of the child's inability to go to the beach that summer. It is often the case that a pleasant image that will occur in the future is a better choice of image than a preferred image from the past that might not occur in the near future.

Autogenic training relies on a cognition to produce the sensation of relaxation. Autogenics are typically combined with another relaxation procedure as a means of enhancing the relaxation effect. Children are asked to repeat certain words, typically "relax" or "calm," as they begin to feel their bodies relaxed and comfortable. With repetition, the word is conditioned to induce a relaxation response. *Meditative breathing* refers to a simple process of controlled breathing. By attending to their inhalation and exhalation, children focus their concentration, which in turn leads to somatic changes and feelings of relaxation. Wexler (1991) has described an imagery-based meditative breathing technique in which the child is asked to imagine 10 candles and then to blow out each candle every time he or she exhales. Such imagery may help keep the child from drifting off during the procedure and possibly to exhale more forcefully in order to "blow out" the candles. *Diaphragmatic breathing* may induce deeper relaxation than meditational breathing. In diaphragmatic breathing, children are taught to breathe from their diaphragm because it induces a deeper state of relaxation than the shallow chest breathing that is often seen when children are asked to breathe in a relaxation procedure. Children often find it difficult to breathe from their diaphragm. One technique that helps teach children this procedure is to ask children to rest a hand on their stomachs and notice the hand rise and fall when breathing is done correctly.

Progressive muscle relaxation is the most common relaxation technique. This procedure involves tensing and relaxing the muscle groups of the body in order to teach the child the difference between a tensed and relaxed muscular state. This procedure also helps children concentrate their attention in order to induce relaxation. Although easy to teach and learn, many children find this technique boring. Therefore, abbreviated procedures that focus on only a few muscle groups have been advocated for children (Beidel & Turner, 1998). In addition, imagery-based progressive muscle relaxation techniques have been developed (e.g., Koeppen, 1974; Ollendick & Cerny, 1981). Koeppen (1974) describes a technique in which imagery is associated with each muscle group. For example, to tense and relax muscles on the face, children imagine that a fly has landed on their nose and they need to get it off by "scrunching up" their nose and face. Shoulders are tensed by asking children to imagine they are turtles pulling their heads into their shell. Leg muscles are tensed by imagining "squishing" feet in mud. These adaptations of progressive muscle relaxation help to engage the children in the procedure. If children develop their own images for each muscle group, engagement may be enhanced even further.

Preparing the Child for a Relaxation Procedure

When working with children, it is especially important to prepare the child for the relaxation technique that will follow. A rationale for the use of relaxation in their particular situation and how it will help their particular symptoms should be outlined. This explanation should include parents so that they, too, understand the rationale. In addition, parents can help explain the procedure to their children and point out to the therapist any parts of the description that might have confused or bothered the child.

The most important part of preparing a child is to develop the correct combination and sequence of relaxation procedures that are best suited to the child. The following procedure, described previously by Powers and Spirito (1998), may be helpful. First, ask the child to make a fist, hold it tightly, and feel the tension in the forearm for about 10 seconds. Then relax the arms by opening the fingers of the hand. Ask the child how it feels after relaxing the arm and to describe the feeling in the hand and arm. Most children need assistance in describing the feeling in their arm. Potential adjectives include tingling, warm or cold, and heavy or light. These questions are used to determine whether the progressive muscle relaxation procedure was pleasant and also to help select the words the child uses to describe a pleasant and relaxed state. These adjectives are then used in the relaxation procedure that follows.

Second, ask the child to shut his or her eyes and to imagine a feeling of relaxation that starts in the fingertips, moves slowly up the fingers, and makes the muscles of the fingers and hands feel (pick the adjectives the child has chosen in the first procedure described above, e.g., warm, tingly). After this procedure, which lasts 10 to 20 seconds, ask the child if he or she was able to imagine the sensations and if he or she has any words to describe the sensation. Then ask the child which technique—the imagery-based or progressive muscle relaxation—feels better. Based on the child's response, the preferred technique is selected for the relaxation procedure. When working with pediatric patients, there will be instances when progressive muscle relaxation will be inappropriate, for example, when working with children with musculoskeletal disorders.

Third, ask the child to take a deep breath and hold it. Observe how long the child is able to comfortably hold his or her breath in order to gauge the length of time you will ask the child to hold his or her breath in the relaxation procedure. This is especially important to determine in children with pulmonary disorders or complications secondary to a chronic disease.

Fourth, gauge the child's imaging ability by asking the child to shut his or her eyes and describe something, for example, the child's bedroom. Note the level of detail used to describe the room. Ask the child to describe colors in the room as well as details on pictures and posters. Ask the child for his or her favorite color. The ease and completeness with which the child generates images will dictate the degree to which imagery is used in the relaxation procedure.

Finally, ask the child for his or her favorite place. Children often pick a family vacation spot, Disney World, or another amusement park. Action scenes are also often selected as a relaxing image. The greater the child's involvement in the image, whether or not it is active or passive, the better it will be in the relaxation procedure.

Sample Relaxation Procedure

The following procedure integrates the preparatory material discussed above into a relaxation procedure appropriate for most children. Comments about the procedure are included throughout the following passages [in brackets]. This technique has been previously published and is reprinted with permission. The procedure is in italics.[1]

Lie back with your arms at your sides and get yourself in as comfortable a position as you can easily find. (pause) *It helps if you close your eyes.* (pause) *I want you to start by taking a deep breath and holding it . . . feel the tension in your chest as you hold it . . . and then slowly let your breath out. Note the difference between the tension and relaxation.* (repeat twice) [Note: This is a simplified meditative breathing technique.] *Now imagine a feeling that starts in your toes that is warm and relaxing. Imagine that feeling moving slowly past the balls of your feet* (pause), *through the arches of your feet* (pause), *through the entire foot* (pause), *and up past your ankle.*

[Note: If the child has identified a favorite color, an alternative procedure to enhance the imagery-based whole-body relaxation is to ask him or her to imagine that color moving up the body as follows:]

Now I also want you to imagine this feeling of relaxation like a wave of color moving up your body, starting down in your toes with your favorite shade of red [Note: or blue, pink, etc.], *slowly moving up through the balls of your feet* (pause), *the wave moving up past your ankle into your calf muscles* (pause), *all the tension draining away* (pause), *your muscles getting loose and relaxed and moving up now past your knees into your thighs.* (pause) *Just imagine that wave of color moving up, and as that wave hits your thigh muscle, you notice those muscles beginning to feel loose, warm, and relaxed.* [Note: We are assuming that the words used by the child to describe relaxation are warm, loose, relaxed.] (pause) *Just notice now how your lower body is feeling more relaxed and comfortable* (pause), *a pleasant feeling.* (pause)

Now imagine that feeling moving up past your hips into your stomach—that wave of red moving up, all the tension draining away (pause), *muscles loose and relaxed* (pause), *the relaxing feeling moving up into your chest—any pain* [Note: if pain is presenting problem] *or tension, any discomfort just draining away, feeling yourself relaxed*

---

1. This material is taken from "Relaxation Training," by S. Powers and A. Spirito, in N. Alessi, J. T. Coyle, S. Harrison, & S. Eth (Eds.), *Handbook of Child and Adolescent Psychiatry*, Vol. 6, pp. 411–417, 1998, New York: John Wiley & Sons. Copyright 1998 by John Wiley & Sons. Reprinted with permission.

and calm (pause), *and then up into your shoulders—all the tension draining away again. Notice a relaxed feeling as you imagine that wave of red moving through your shoulder muscles* (pause), *down your upper arms* (pause), *relaxed and calm* (pause), *down past your elbows into your forearms—a warm, relaxing feeling.* (pause) *That wave of red moving past your wrists into the palms of your hands, warm and relaxed* (pause), *down to your fingertips, relaxed and calm* (pause), *making your whole body relaxed.*

Now that you've seen how to make your whole body relaxed, we can do the same for your neck and face by just imagining that wave moving up now through your neck muscles (pause), *loose and warm* (pause), *past your chin* (pause), *the wave of red moving up past your lips and nose, all the tension draining away* (pause), *warm and comfortable, as it moves up past your eyes and forehead* (pause), *warm and relaxed, warm and comfortable over the top of your head* (pause), *your whole body is relaxed and calm.*

[Note: It is important to pace the whole-body relaxation procedure so that the child responds most beneficially. As the therapist recites the procedure, he or she can note whether the child stays engaged in the procedure or starts to have difficulty attending to the instructions. If the latter is true, it may be helpful to speed up the process a little bit and not to focus so much on the relaxation in order to maintain the child's attention and interest in the procedure.]

Now that you've made your whole body relaxed and calm, we can improve on these feelings of relaxation in the following way: I want you to just imagine yourself in your bedroom at home and about to walk down the stairs to watch some TV. You're barefoot and the stairs have very thick, deep, comfortable carpeting, and it feels very pleasant on your feet. Walk down the stairs very slowly because it feels so good as you walk through this thick carpeting. (pause) *Count the stairs as you go along* (pause), *and, with each step you count, you'll become more and more relaxed.*

[Note: This procedure is known as a deepening technique and is commonly used in order to achieve a deep state of relaxation during a hypnotic procedure. It is a worthwhile technical addition when working with an attentive child. The assumption here is that this particular child has a bedroom on the second floor. Many children will be able to count exactly the number of stairs they have at home, and the therapist should use this number. There are other ways to use a deepening procedure, such as counting trees on a walk through the forest, or counting waves as one sits on the beach. Once again, in the initial assessment procedure, the therapist must decide whether to use deepening and the best way to use it.]

Count the first step—one—and notice your body getting loose and relaxed. (pause) *Now two, calm and comfortable* (pause), *three, feelings of warmth and relaxation throughout your body.*

[Note: The therapist should continue this procedure, up to the chosen number of steps. There are many guidelines about how to enhance the deepening effect. Some simple ones include maintaining a sufficiently long pause between the numbers and that the tone and the loudness of the voice should vary.]

Now you are about to take your last step, and when you do so, a wave of relaxation will move throughout your entire body and you will feel your whole body totally relaxed and comfortable. And now the last step, ten. Feel that wave of red move up through your entire body as you become totally relaxed and comfortable. (pause) *Now use your imagination and see yourself slowly moving over to a comfortable chair near your TV and taking the remote control. This is a special remote control that shows your own relaxing thoughts and images on the TV. Today your thoughts and images are of calm, relaxing places, the kinds we talked about earlier—being at your grandmother's house.* [Note: Or going to the beach, etc.—the child's chosen images are described.] *The images will come on the TV.* (pause) *You can control the image with your thoughts.* (pause) *Try to stay on one image for a little while, but you can switch images if you find one more relaxing. Just use your imagination for the next few moments.* (pause) *As you do so, notice how your body becomes more and more relaxed.*

[Note: This imagery-based procedure is directed by the child. The length of time the therapist allows the child to engage in the imagery varies, depending on the child's age and involvement in the relaxation procedure up to this point. However, it is better for the child to use the image in a short period of silence rather than too long a period during which time the child becomes distracted. In most cases, 30 seconds is long enough for this type of technique. Because this technique is self-directed, external noises and internal thoughts can disrupt the relaxation procedure very easily. Thus, it is also helpful to use a statement such as the following before the child starts the self-directed imagery.]

While you are relaxing, if you hear any noises they will not bother you. (pause) *Just let them fade in and out* (pause), *in and out, as you continue to focus on your relaxing image.* (pause) *If you have any thoughts that seem to distract you, just let them fade in and out, in and out, as you focus on this relaxing, calm image.* (pause) *Let's do so for the next few moments, being very relaxed and calm.*

The therapist can end the relaxation procedure with the following statement:

Now that you have been able to make yourself very relaxed and calm, you can count silently to yourself from 5 down to 1, and when you reach 1 you will feel alert and refreshed, almost as if you've taken a pleasant nap, and you can return to any activities feeling relaxed and comfortable and calm.

[Note: The therapist counts, slowly (and silently) from 5 down to 1 and observes how slowly the child counts from 5 down to 1.]

An alternative ending to this procedure can be used for children with sleep problems. In cases in which the child might use this tape during the day and also at night, the following statement can be added:

Now you have a choice; if you'd like (pause), *you can drift off to sleep, a deep, peaceful, relaxing sleep* (pause), *or, if you prefer, you can count from 5 down to 1.* (Repeat the above procedure.)

Problem-Solving Methods

Problem solving is a commonly used technique in treatments for children and adolescents. Problem-solving procedures are used to address problems related to limited flexibility, generating alternative solutions, and ability to identify positive consequences of potential solutions. Although there are several different approaches to problem-solving training, the SOLVE system, described below, covers the basic steps and has been used with adolescents (Donaldson, Spirito, & Overholser, 2003).[2]

We're going to review with you a method for solving problems. We call it the S-O-L-V-E system. Each letter in the word "SOLVE" stands for a different step of the problem-solving process. As you can see on the card, "S" stands for "select a problem." The first step in solving a problem is to identify what the problem is. The second step is "O" or "options." After you identify the problem, you need to make a list of ALL of the possible options—not just the ones you think would work. The bigger the list you make, the better the chance you have of solving the problem! The next step in the problem-solving process is "L" or "likely outcomes." You need to take the list you made up and decide what might happen when you try each of these options. You can rate them in terms of whether you think things would get better or worse with each option. Then, you would narrow down your list to one option and pick the "very best one" to do. Then you try it out, and at the end, you "evaluate" or decide whether or not the problem still exists. If it does, you

---

2. This procedure is taken from pp. 305–307 of "Treatment of Adolescent Suicide Attempters," by D. Donaldson, A. Spirito, and J. Overholser, in A. Spirito & J. Overholser (Eds.), *Evaluating and Treating Adolescent Suicide Attempters: From Research to Practice*, pp. 295–321, 2003, New York: Academic Press. Copyright 2003 by Academic Press. Adapted with permission from Elsevier.

go back to your options, weigh them out, and pick the next very best one to try. You keep doing this until your problem is solved. (Adolescent repeats the steps.) *Let's try it.*

After problem-solving skills are successfully taught, treatment can address the presenting problem and other subsequent problems using the same system. Often, the adolescent will have initial difficulties generating options. The therapist may need to model the skills in order to help the adolescent learn these new behaviors. Similarly, cognitive distortions may be elicited while generating "likely outcomes," which can then be addressed. An example of utilizing the SOLVE system is as follows:

Think of a problem that brought you here. What was that? (pause) *That's great. You've accomplished the first step in solving a problem, which is to identify what the problem is. Do you remember the second step?* (Prompt: *What does it start with? What does "O" stand for?*)

That's right. You need to think of as many things that a person faced with that problem could possibly do in that situation. That includes options you think would work as well as options you don't think would work so well.

Wait for the adolescent to generate as many options as he or she can. When the child stops, prompt for more by saying, *You've thought of some already. Keep listing as many as you possibly can.*

When the child stops again, state, *Great! You actually made me think of one,* and share another example with the adolescent, being careful to indicate which option you generated versus those that were generated by the adolescent. Some adolescents will only generate options that they perceive to be workable solutions. The therapist can prompt the adolescent to generate a minimum of at least two strategies he or she thinks would work as well as two strategies that he or she thinks might not work very well.

You generated several options. What is the next step? (Prompt: *What does it start with? What does "L" stand for?*)

That's right. Now you need to weigh each option and decide whether you think it would or would not be a helpful option. Let's take the first option you listed, (state that here). *Do you think this is something that would or would not help in that situation? Rate each one either positive, negative, or positive and negative depending upon how helpful you expect it to be.*

What's the next step of solving the problem? (Prompt: *What does it start with? What does "V" stand for?*) *That's right. You have to pick the very best one to do from your list of options. Which would you pick?*

When the adolescent responds ask, *What is the last step of problem solving?* (Prompt: *What does it start with? What does "E" stand for?*)

Yes, "evaluate," or go back and see how it turned out. If your problem still exists, then you need to go back to your list of options and pick a different one. If your problem is solved, then you don't have to do anything.

When appropriate, the clinician can also illustrate the presenting problem (e.g., noncompliance with medication) as a failure in problem solving using the system:

What would happen if you only had one option listed and you tried that and it didn't help your problem?

Cover up all but one option from the list the child generated and wait for a response.

Yes. You'd be stuck. That's kind of like what happened when you decided not to take your medication when you were out with your friends. You didn't feel like you had many options, you felt pretty stuck, so you picked the only option you thought you had, which was to not stop and take your meds. That's why we've found "SOLVE" to be helpful to adolescents who have been in that situation. The more you practice coming up with a list of options and the more options you have to choose from when you have a problem, the less likely you'll feel stuck or there's nothing you can do.

Anger Control

Pediatric psychologists frequently encounter situations in which children are frustrated and angry about uncontrollable medical events. Some of these children and adolescents may benefit from training designed to lower arousal. Affect regulation techniques that are used in cognitive therapy include training adolescents to recognize stimuli that provoke negative emotions and learning to reduce physiological arousal via self-talk and relaxation.

Feindler and Ecton (1986) developed a system of cognitive mediation techniques and arousal reduction methods to help adolescents with anger control problems. These methods may be useful for some medical patients. In their system, Feindler and Ecton use the acronym CALMDOWN to summarize the eight cognitive and behavioral skills taught in their program. Adolescents are first taught "*c*ues" for identifying anger triggers and to prepare for provocation. Adolescents are then taught to "*a*lter" the thoughts that lead to the angry feelings. In the next phase of the protocol, the goal is to "*let*" the adolescent use self-statements to guide them through angry provocations. Behavioral strategies are also introduced, including relaxation techniques to "*modulate*" physiologic arousal, and adolescents are "*directed*" to communicate more effectively and act out assertively, rather than aggressively, in conflict situations. "*Organization*" of the anger-control process is taught using problem-solving training. "*Working*" through the protocol via modeling and behavioral rehearsal is followed by "*negotiating*" a commitment to use the newly taught skills in anger-provoking situations. After receiving this self-instruction training, the goal is for adolescents to repeat calming statements to themselves during interpersonal conflicts and use relaxation techniques to minimize affective arousal.

Donaldson et al. (2003) provide the following guidelines for clinicians when incorporating affect management into treatment. First, present a rationale for affect management training. For example, the therapist might point out to the teen that he or she often feels angry or out of control and that such feelings of distress are not uncommon among his or her peers. The therapist should then go on to explain that there are some techniques that may prove useful in gaining better control of emotions. It is also important to clearly explain the relationship between the adolescent's thoughts and his/her bodily reactions—that is, explain that negative thoughts about a situation will lead to feelings of anger, frustration, or irritation. These feelings in turn result in certain physiological reactions that vary across persons. Elicit from the adolescent his/her most characteristic physical reaction (e.g., stomach upset, sweating, heart racing, etc.). Make sure the adolescent understands that the longer he or she maintains the negative thought, the more physically tense he or she will become, and in turn, the more likely these feelings of tension will result in some sort of outburst. Therefore, the key to controlling this negative sequence of events is to control one's thoughts. One good way to describe this sequence of events is to use the example of a match setting off a firecracker (Feindler & Ecton, 1986). One might encounter this type of reaction in a hospitalized adolescent upset with hospital staff for intruding on his or her privacy. The therapist might discuss how a nurse coming into the room to give the patient another pill starts this chain of events. The therapist should elicit the negative thoughts that arise when the nurse enters the room and the corresponding emotions and body tension that accompany these thoughts. The therapist should then focus on how changing these negative thoughts can short-circuit this process and reduce chances of an angry outburst.

Cognitive Coping Skills Training

Cognitive coping skills training has been used with children for a variety of presenting problems, including anxiety, impulse control, and depression. The techniques used for anxious children may have greatest applicability for children in medical settings. Stress inoculation, one specific procedure, based on a cognitive model of self-control postulated by Meichenbaum (1976), focuses on altering the internal dialogue of the child. The treatment protocol occurs in three phases: (a) conceptualization, (b) skills acquisition and rehearsal, and (c) application and follow-through. This procedure is briefly described here because it can be applied to many anxiety-provoking situations encountered in the medical setting. A more detailed discussion of the procedure can be found in Grace, Spirito, Finch, and Ott (1993).

After establishing rapport with the child and presenting an understandable rationale and explanation for the procedure, behavioral and cognitive methods are taught to the child. The child is instructed on how to identify early signs of anxiety that in turn serve as a signal to perform a coping response. The two main techniques used in this protocol are an abbreviated relaxation procedure and self-instruction. Only the latter is described here.

The following approach (adapted from Grace et al., 1993[3]) might be used for a fearful child in the hospital.

Lots of people, both kids and grownups, can get scared when they are in the hospital alone. So I'm going to teach you how to be less scared.

For young children, reinforce their efforts with material reinforcers: *If you can try your best, I have some prizes over here and you can choose one when you're done.*

[Note: If the child says, "I'm not afraid, so I don't have to do this," then the therapist might respond, "This will probably be easy for you. If you try and do your best to follow directions, when you're done you can choose a small prize from my grab bag."]

Let me tell you a few things about being afraid. When people are afraid, they say things to themselves like, "There will be no one here to watch me if my mother leaves

---

3. This material is adapted from Grace et al. in A. J. Finch, W. M. Nelson, & E. Ott (Eds.), *Cognitive-Behavioral Procedures With Children and Adolescents: A Practical Guide*, 1993, Boston: Allyn & Bacon. Copyright 1993 by Pearson Education. Reprinted/adapted with permission.

my hospital room even for a few minutes. Something bad could happen to me" or "My doctor is not working tonight and I don't know the other doctors."

So you see, when people are afraid they say lots of scared things to themselves. And you know what happens when you say these things to yourself? You get even more scared. What sort of scared things do you say to yourself when you are alone in the hospital?

[Note: Young children usually have difficulty generating self-statements. It sometimes helps to ask them to "run a movie" through their head about the last time they were alone in the hospital.]

When people are scared, sometimes their bodies do funny things, too. For some kids, their stomach starts to feel funny, other kids feel shaky or sweaty, and other kids start to breathe fast.

Now do you know what people who are not afraid say to themselves? They say things like, "It's okay, my mother will be back soon. I can talk with the kid next to me and his mom. The nurse knows my mom is gone, and she will look after me. If I need to talk to my mom, I can always call her."

Saying these things help to keep kids from getting too scared. So here's what we're going to do today. We're going to teach you to say the right things to yourself so you won't be afraid.

In the next phase of the protocol, the therapist models how to use self-statements (and relaxation) for the child's presenting problems:

Okay, now I'm going to show you how you can use what I taught you to keep calm in the hospital when you're alone. I'm going to pretend that I'm alone in the hospital room. I want you to listen to what I say, and if you can tell me some of the things I said after I'm done, you'll get to choose a prize.

Verbal self-instructions are first modeled by the therapist and then rehearsed by the child. The verbalizations are generally of four types. First, defining the problem is used to help children guide themselves as to what they should do and say in a specific anxiety-provoking situation. For example, a child who is anxious about staying alone in the hospital might say, "What should I do when I'm scared because my mother is not here? I know I need to do things to make me feel it's okay to be alone in the hospital." Second, the child needs to focus his or her attention on the coping task at hand, for example, "I have to concentrate and remember to do what I practiced when I'm alone in the hospital." Third, the child is instructed to use the coping statements that have been developed in training, for example, "I'm starting to feel nervous, I'd better take a deep breath and relax." And fourth, the child rewards himself or herself for engaging in the coping process.

In the next phase of the protocol, the child performs the task out loud and the therapist instructs and prompts use of self-statements. After some practice, the prompting is faded and the child is asked to use the self-statements out loud without guidance. Future sessions are used to fade from "out loud" speech to whispers to covert self-instructions. After each of these different sessions, the therapist rewards the child for his or her efforts and asks the child to make his or her own self-reinforcing statements.

This procedure can be adapted to many problems, performed over time in multiple sessions, or condensed into even one session if the situation demands quick action. It is important to prepare the child for relapse and to understand that "slipping" will happen but that he or she will be able to get back under control with some renewed practice.

Helpful Hints

There are any number of situational and individual factors that will make implementation of the cognitive and behavioral procedures described here less than ideal. A number of recommendations that may be useful in implementing these procedures, taken primarily from Friedberg, Crosby, Friedberg, Rutter, and Knight (2000) and Grace et al. (1993), are presented below.

1. Therapists must be flexible in determining the rate at which a child can incorporate the material. Some children may also be embarrassed stating their thoughts aloud.
2. Therapist reinforcement should be gradually faded as the child becomes more facile at self-reinforcement. Response-cost procedures may prove more effective for some children than direct reinforcement. The therapeutic relationship is critically important in helping to maintain the child's interest in the task.
3. When modeling cognitive coping, include negative self-statements that are corrected with positive self-statements.
4. Because many children have trouble generating self-statements, the therapist should provide a large number of self-statements from which the child can select. Most children, however, settle on one or two self-statements. Self-generated statements are typically the best statements.

5. Make sure the self-statements are practiced in real-life situations under conditions of affective arousal in order to enhance maintenance and generalization.
6. For most children, booster sessions are needed because the effects of training diminish over time.
7. Teach parents the basics of cognitive coping so that they can reinforce these procedures with the child. Having the child teach these skills to another child is another way to increase generalization and maintenance.

Conclusions

This chapter has reviewed common cognitive and behavioral techniques used in treatment protocols deemed effective with children. Adaptations should be made as needed to best apply these techniques to pediatric patients.

4 Multiperson and Systemic Interventions

There are compelling reasons to treat children with pediatric health concerns in the context of their families, first and foremost, and also in other essential systems, such as hospitals and schools. Although the importance of interpersonal and family approaches in pediatric health is theoretically and intuitively apparent, the literature on family and other systemic interventions in psychology generally is at an earlier stage of development than that on individual approaches.

In this chapter we provide a general background on the history and rationale for a family and systems focus in pediatric psychology interventions, including a summary of major categories of family intervention. We then review empirical evidence for existing family, group, and other systemic interventions. This literature cuts across disease entities and disciplinary boundaries. Since family interventions have their roots in many different schools of family theory and therapy, it is not possible in this chapter to present a concise summary of relevant family intervention approaches.[1] Rather, we present a discussion of conceptual and methodological issues impacting future multiperson intervention research. This chapter concludes with a "case study" of a manualized intervention that integrates family and cognitive-behavioral treatment approaches.

---

1. More information about general schools of family therapy may be obtained in recent textbooks. For example, see R. Mikesell, D. D. Lusterman, and S. McDaniel, *Integrating Family Therapy: Handbook of Family Psychology and Systems Theory* (1995); M. Nichols and R. Schwartz, *Essentials of Family Therapy* (2004); and D. Waters and E. W. Lawrence, *Courage, Competence, and Change: An Approach to Family Therapy* (1993). Other sources of information about family therapy include peer-reviewed journals such as the *Journal of Family Psychology, Family Process,* and *Families, Systems, and Health.*

The Child in a Systemic Context

Children grow and develop in social contexts. The study of children in context has a long tradition and one that is readily applicable to pediatric psychology intervention. Most children seek health care because their family members initiate it. Although the child's or adolescent's consent (or assent) for medical treatment is important, full responsibility for agreeing to treatment and following through with treatment recommendations and implications rests with the family (generally, but not always, parents). Interventions that either focus on family members or the family as a whole or incorporate others in a child-oriented intervention make intuitive sense and have empirical support. Thinking beyond the family and the immediate hospital setting is also essential. Indeed, even patients with serious and chronic pediatric illnesses spend increasingly little time in the hospital, necessitating interventions that link patient, family, hospital, communities, and, perhaps most prominently, schools (Power, DuPaul, Shapiro, & Kazak, 2003).

Social ecology is a model that has been applied to understanding the systemic nature of pediatric illness and offers a well-accepted and helpful framework for conceptualizing and providing treatment (Kazak, 1989; Kazak, Rourke, & Crump, 2003). Based on the work of developmental psychologist Urie Bronfenbrenner (1979), social ecology views children embedded within a series of spheres of influence, each with its own social systems (figure 4.1). Most pediatric psychology research and practice occur within the innermost circle, at the level of the individual child with a specific disease, and may include members of the immediate family system. More distal circles in this model encourage consideration of the reciprocal impact of other systems on children. Certainly for children with pediatric health conditions, health care, peer, school, and neighborhood ecologies are prominent. The impact of broader systems is undeniably important for these children, as well as for their families. For example, special education and family leave legislation, and their interpretation and implementation, can have dramatic effects. Similarly, social ecology emphasizes the important context of culture and subcultures. Family beliefs and behaviors are influenced heavily by ethnicity, social class, and family structure. This highlights the complexity of conceptualizing and implementing effective interventions in the face of many sources of variability. Yet it also underscores the importance of recognizing and utilizing contextually valid approaches.

A social ecological perspective is highly congruent with intervention in pediatric psychology because it rests on theories of development. That is, children

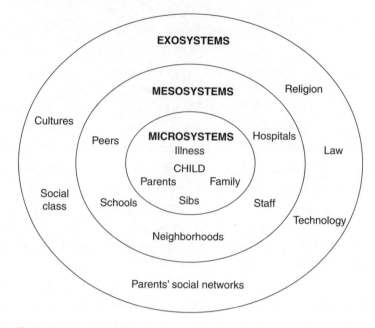

Figure 4.1   Social ecology views children embedded within a series of spheres of influence, each with its own social system.

grow and develop through their interactions with others in important social contexts. Most research on pediatric populations has occurred at the level of the family system, arguably the most important system in the lives of young children. By conceptualizing change at the level of the family, we have the opportunity to change the context in which children live and develop, thereby ideally maximizing the child's outcome and also that of other important people in the child's life.

History of Family Intervention With Pediatric Populations

Psychology was a relative latecomer in the area of families and illness. For example, social work services in hospitals have been an accepted part of care for many years, whereas psychologists entered the general area of health subsequent to World War II and largely provided psychological testing at that time (Starr, 1982). Similarly, the early years of family therapy (the 1950s and 1960s) were influenced heavily by psychiatrists, who argued for an alternative to psychodynamic treatments that would affect the patient in the context of family. Their focus, however, was primarily on mental health conditions, often the more severe psychopathologies. Social workers and psychiatrists provided clinical care but generally without conducting research on effectiveness. Family social scientists, largely based in sociology or human development, conducted research on basic family patterns associated with medical conditions and developed educational and preventive programs.

There are rich clinical perspectives from the field of family therapy that are an important part of the history of family intervention in pediatrics. Minuchin and colleagues explored the important idea that family functioning might affect the course of treatment for childhood diseases such as asthma and diabetes. Using structural family therapy, they selected a small group of children with diabetes, asthma, and anorexia nervosa who had not responded successfully to their previous medical and mental health treatments (Minuchin et al., 1975; Minuchin, Rosman, & Baker, 1978). Their hypothesis was that the life-threatening symptoms that emerged from poor adherence to medical treatments (e.g., severe asthma attacks, ketoacidosis, dramatic weight loss) served to mask underlying conflicts among family members. The effort to describe the role of family intervention and to offer family-based treatments was influential, although not subsequently evaluated.

The influence of structural family therapy and the Minuchin et al. (1978) groundwork is evident in more recent work by Beatrice Wood and her colleagues in the biobehavioral family model. Wood (1995) introduced the idea of biobehavioral reactivity to describe how interpersonal processes in the family may influence disease activity in families of children with Crohn's disease, ulcerative colitis, functional recurrent abdominal pain, and moderate to severe asthma (Miller & Wood, 1994; Wood et al., 1989). More recently, this group has shown that attachment styles between mothers and children can mediate the relationship between functional health status and depressive symptoms in the child (Bleil, Ramesh, Miller, & Wood, 2000).

Based on the biopsychosocial model (Engel, 1977), medical family therapy provides a model of intervention that targets individuals and families who are affected by an illness by showing that "all problems are at once, biological, psychological, and social" (McDaniel, Hepworth, & Doherty, 1992). Central to medical family therapy is a collaborative, multidisciplinary approach, with family therapists working directly with other health care providers to treat the multiple components of the medical problem. This model has been used primarily in family practice and is prominently reflected in the Collaborative Family Healthcare Association (www.cfha.org) and in the journal *Families, Systems, and Health*.

Evidence-Based Family Interventions in Pediatric Psychology

Family intervention is highly relevant across many common pediatric issues and patient groups. While family interventions are often discussed as if they were one type of intervention, it is important to distinguish among the various types, including therapy, psychoeducation, information and support, and direct service (Campbell & Patterson, 1995). Each differs in its goals, approaches, and outcomes. The majority of family intervention studies in pediatric psychology fall into the category of therapy or psychoeducation. That is, they are therapy in the sense of reducing symptoms or augmenting specific outcomes, or are psychoeducational, emphasizing the provision of information (e.g., knowledge about sickle cell disease or diabetes and general principles for management) or teaching specific skills to accomplish increased competence in medical management.

Our review of these interventions includes treatments that focus on an individual member of the family (e.g., mothers) and dyads within the family (e.g., parent–child, parents), as well as those that are directed toward the family as a whole. We have also included interventions that treat multiple members of the family (e.g., parents and children separately). While not necessarily recognized as family interventions from a conceptual point of view, they target family members in the course of intervention.

Adherence

Barriers to treatment adherence for pediatric patients are a well-known area of concern and include well-established treatments for the individual child (see chapter 6). However, parents are key in how treatment recommendations are implemented and must necessarily monitor this process. Characteristics of the parents and the family are also likely to have an impact on the outcome of efforts to improve adherence. Interventions with multiple members of the family related to adherence are available for patients with cystic fibrosis, diabetes, and obesity.

Given the large literature on adherence in diabetes, it is not surprising to find that interventions with this patient population are among the most advanced in their inclusion of families. Using a 6-week multifamily model for adolescents with diabetes and their families, Satin, La Greca, Zigo, and Skyler (1989) provided evidence for the importance of family support in adherence. Their treatment protocol included essential elements associated with adherence, such as communication skills, problem solving, and support for self-care. It also included a creative family "simulation" of diabetes. In the simulation, the adolescents "taught" their parents to manage diabetes care and administered injections of normal saline, using simulated glucose readings to suggest alterations in their eating, exercise, and blood tests. The exercise provided families with the opportunity to change roles in the management of diabetes, one intended to enhance communication and appreciation for the difficulty of parent and teen roles.

Particularly with adolescents, issues related to adherence often involve patterns of parent–adolescent conflict that are normative developmentally but accentuated by the pressures to achieve optimal control of the diabetes. Behavioral family systems therapy (BFST) has been compared both to standard treatment and to an education and support condition in adolescents with diabetes (Wysocki et al., 2000). BFST provided a means by which both general and diabetes-related family conflict could be reduced, although this was not strongly associated with diabetes control or adherence. BFST has recently been evaluated in cystic fibrosis (Quittner et al., 2000), an important step in establishing commonalities in adherence treatments across and within illnesses.

Anderson and her team developed a 20- to 30-minute brief teamwork intervention directed toward preventing the increase in conflict typically seen during the early adolescent years related to diabetes care (Anderson, Brackett, Ho, & Laffel, 2000). The intervention appeared to stem the expected increase in parent–adolescent conflict that was seen in the comparison group. A subsequent randomized clinical trial compared a family-focused teamwork intervention to standard multidisciplinary diabetes care in order to assess the impact of the intervention on glycemic control and adherence (Laffel et al., 2003). The content of the two study arms was identical, but the teamwork intervention group received coaching on the importance of the parent–child dyad in diabetes management and ended each session with a written plan for sharing responsibility for the different facets of the diabetes regimen. The positive outcomes seen in terms of increased glycemic control was attributed to increased parental involvement in diabetes care in a way that reflected collaborative relationships and seemed to avoid increases in parent–child conflict (Laffel et al., 2003).

The concept of working within a family-centered model to affect medical care and adherence in diabetes is further seen in another randomized clinical trial from this group (Svoren, Butler, Levine, Anderson, & Laffel, 2003). Children and adolescents with diabetes and their families were randomized to one of three arms. In the care ambassador (CA) arm, a research assistant worked with the family to arrange appointments, tracked appointment attendance, and offered to facilitate help with billing or other questions about their medical care. In the CA+ condition, a psychoeducational intervention was also provided by the CA. The third condition, standard care, did not receive CA support or psychoeducational materials. Families in the CA and CA+ arms had better attendance for medical appointments, but the relationship with glycemic control was limited to those patients who initially had higher risks involved in diabetic control (Svoren et al., 2003). Evidence for reduced medical expenses was seen for the patients in the CA+ group. This intervention provides support for the importance of focusing resources on those families at greatest need and also shows the success of a relatively low-intensity intervention on multiple outcomes.

Stark (2000, 2003) has developed a behavioral group treatment approach for 4- to 12-year-old children with cystic fibrosis and their parents in order to achieve higher rates of adherence to a high-energy, high-fat diet to treat pancreatic insufficiency. In the treatment program entitled Behavioral Intervention for Change Around Growth and Energy (Be in CHARGE!), parents and patients are treated separately using a protocol that emphasizes nutritional information, calorie goals, and developmentally appropriate approaches for food intake of targeted foods. The techniques used are standard behavioral approaches (e.g., praise, reward, ignoring, shaping). A series of reports established the efficacy of the intervention (weight gain), with children serving as their own controls (Stark, Bowen, Tyc, Evans, & Passero, 1990; Stark et al., 1993) and contrasted with wait-list control (Stark et al., 1996). In a study comparing Be in CHARGE! with a nutrition education condition, preliminary data supported increases in energy intake by the treatment group (Stark et al., 2003).

With regard to weight management and obesity, the involvement of the family is widely seen as critical in altering the environmental context to support the difficult behavioral changes necessary for weight loss (Marcus, Levine, & Kalarchian, 2003). Indeed, behavioral treatment for childhood obesity that focuses on eating and exercise behaviors in both parents and children has been shown to be effective in long-term child weight reduction (i.e., 2 years) and diminished child behavior problems. Further, when this treatment is expanded to incorporate problem-solving training, over time improvements in parents' distress have been observed (Epstein, Paluch, Gordy, Saelens, & Ernst, 2000). Recent experimental work on pharmacologic approaches to pediatric obesity also support the inclusion of behavioral therapy that includes separate group treatments for parents and patients (Berkowitz, Wadden, Tershakovec, & Cronquist, 2003).

Disease Knowledge and Management

Another area of potential importance for interventions with families concerns education about diseases and treatments. Given the complexity of many treatment protocols, mastery of knowledge about illnesses and their treatments is important and can be targeted toward the family, rather than focused on the child (patient). For example, in sickle cell disease, a family psychoeducational approach integrating biological (e.g., knowledge about sickle cell disease), psychological (e.g., psychological symptoms, cognitive functioning), and sociocultural (e.g., racial identity, family resources) issues was contrasted with standard sickle cell education (Kaslow et al., 2000). The psychoeducational family approach was associated with increased knowledge about sickle cell disease for both children and parents; for child participants, enhanced disease knowledge was maintained over time (6 months). A particular strength of this work is its thoughtful development of the intervention in terms of cultural sensitivity, an essential component in joining with families to enhance their competence in providing medical care for their children (Kaslow & Brown, 1995).

Reducing Distress

Interventions to address the distress experienced by one or more members of the family are particularly compelling because of the well-established strain and psychological distress for family members (particularly parents) associated with having an ill child. However, relatively few intervention studies have been conducted in this area. One likely complicating factor is overall general positive psychological adjustment of parents and families. That is, although stressful, most families who have children with pediatric illnesses are basically adaptive "average" functioning families. Therefore, they may not be motivated to engage in treatment studies that may be more appropriate for those whose distress is more clinically palpable.

On a related note, even significant distress may dissipate over time, regardless of intervention. For example, Hoekstra-Weebers, Heuval, Jaspers, Kamps, and Klip (1998) evaluated a psychoeducational intervention for parents of children newly diagnosed with cancer. They found that parental well-being improved in both groups over time. Similarly, in a brief stress inoculation intervention focused on mothers of children undergoing bone marrow transplantation, mothers in the intervention condition did not differ in their outcomes from the control condition, with both groups showing improvement, although indications in support of specific timing for intervention (e.g., prior to admission for transplantation) were suggested in the data (Streisand, Rodrigue, Houck, Graham-Pole, & Berlant, 2000).

In general, stronger support has emerged for family interventions when they have more highly focused outcomes rather than general ones (Kazak, 2005). For example, in two multisite randomized clinical trials of an eight-session intervention using maternal problem solving in mothers of children with cancer, a pilot study ($N = 92$) and a subsequent larger trial ($N = 430$) showed that problem solving around specific situations related to the child's treatment was more effective than treatment as usual in reducing negative affectivity while also enhancing problem-solving skills (Sahler et al., 2002, 2005).

Across members of the families of teenage survivors of childhood cancer (survivors, mothers, fathers, adolescent siblings), there is support for posttraumatic stress symptoms (PTSS) as significant and distressing sequelae of experiencing a life-threatening illness and its treatment (Alderfer, Labay, & Kazak, 2003; R. Brown, Madan-Swain, & Lambert, 2003; Kazak et al., 1997, 2001; Kazak, Alderfer, Rourke, et al., 2004; Manne, DuHamel, Gallelli, Sorgen, & Redd, 1998; Manne et al., 2002). An intervention that integrates cognitive-behavioral and family therapy approaches, entitled the Surviving Cancer Competently Intervention Program (SCCIP; Kazak et al., 1999), has been developed. The results of a randomized clinical trial of 151 adolescent cancer survivors indicate that the SCCIP treatment was more effective than a wait-list control condition in reducing symptoms of arousal in survivors and cancer-related intrusive thoughts for fathers (Kazak, Alderfer, Streisand, et al., 2004). An adaptation of SCCIP for parents and caregivers of children newly diagnosed with cancer (SCCIP-ND) has been developed and is currently being evaluated in a randomized clinical trial. By intervening at the time of diagnosis, the intent is to provide a preventative approach to the development of PTSS. Initial pilot data support the feasibility of providing this intervention at diagnosis (Kazak, Simms, et al., in press). The SCCIP protocol for families of adolescent cancer survivors is discussed in more detail later in this chapter.

Other Family Outcomes

In addition to focusing on disease-related outcomes or specific symptoms of patients and parents, interventions may be directed toward outcomes related to other members of the family system. Given concern about the impact of pediatric illness on marital relationships and on the healthy siblings in the family, interventions addressing these outcomes are important.

Emotionally focused therapy (EFT), which targets a couple's negative patterns of interaction and attachment bond, has been shown to reduce marital distress in families of chronically ill children; improvements were stable over a 2-year period (J. Walker, Johnson, Manion, & Cloutier, 1996). The EFT model offers an opportunity to examine not only how the marital relationship is affected by the illness but also how the disease course and the child's functioning are influenced by the marital relationship.

A recent meta-analysis of studies related to sibling adjustment in pediatric psychology concluded that there was a modest negative effect for siblings, particularly when their sibling's illness had a notable impact on daily family functioning (Sharpe & Rossiter, 2002). The review also highlighted differences in the perspectives of parents and siblings in terms of psychological adjustment, consistent with other comparisons of parent and child reports. In general, parents express concerns about their healthy children, but little research attention has been devoted to intervention in this area.

There have been a handful of interesting pilot studies related to sibling group interventions. Although based on small, nonrandom samples and using uncontrolled designs, they offer preliminary support for the importance of further work in this area. Three quite similar studies pertain to siblings of children with cancer. Dolgin, Somer, Zaidel, and Zaizov (1997) reported that siblings had fewer interpersonal problems, less preoccupation with their brother's or sister's illness, improved knowledge of cancer, and more positive mood after a six-session sibling group. Similarly, siblings completing an 8-week program showed declines in self-report indices of depression, anxiety, and fear of disease (Barrera, Chung, Greenberg, & Fleming, 2002). And a five-session sibling intervention resulted in less anxiety for siblings (Houtzager, Grootenhuis, & Last, 2001). In a group intervention with siblings of children representing a range of pediatric health problems, Lobato and Kao (2001) showed similar improvements in knowledge and adjustment, gains that were maintained at a 3-month follow-up.

Group Interventions in Pediatric Psychology

The most well-known and effective interventions involving group approaches are those (noted above) related to the use of patient and parent groups for adherence and weight management. Surprisingly little research has evaluated other types of group interventions in pediatric psychology. While the logistics of providing group treatment in general may impede efforts to develop effective group treatment programs, the possibility of drawing on peer relationships to address a range of concerns related to pediatric illness is clearly important. In reviewing the literature in this area, Plante, Lobato, and Engel (2001) concluded that there was insufficient development of this research to provide evidence for the effectiveness of emotional support groups or psychoeducational groups.

Social skills interventions are one of the more promising areas for group intervention. A social skills training intervention for children with cancer was contrasted with a school reintegration program and showed some evidence for improved social skills over a 9-month period (Varni, Katz, Colegrove, & Dolgin, 1993). More recently, a social skills intervention was piloted in a small group of children with brain tumors, with evidence for improvements in functioning (Barakat et al., 2003).

A creative intervention was developed and piloted by Greco, Pendley, McDonell, and Reeves (2001) incorporated friends of adolescents with diabetes ($n = 21$ pairs) in four 2-hour sessions that included presentations, handouts, activities, and homework, with the goals of integrating friends into teens' management of diabetes. Preliminary pre- and postintervention data showed improvements in knowledge and peer support, and parents reported improvements in family conflicts related to diabetes care.

Other Systemic Interventions in Pediatric Psychology

Guided by systemic models, interventions with systems other than the family are necessary in order to have a truly ecological impact on pediatric health care. Conceptually, the integration of health care, family, school, and community systems is essential in providing comprehensive integrated care that addresses the many concerns of families of ill children (Power et al., 2003).

School settings are perhaps the most obvious for interventions related to child health, because they afford the opportunity to address a range of concerns, especially those related to academic and social functioning. Most interventions in schools have been based on the concept of school "reintegration." That is, as children newly diagnosed with a serious illness (e.g., cancer) return to school after initial diagnosis and treatment, a program of education and support can help facilitate the child's return to school. Ideally, the child and family feel more secure in knowing that the school is ready to have the child back in the classroom, the child's peers are prepared for differences in how the child may look or act, and the teachers have had the opportunity to establish communication with the hospital and family about the child's condition. There is a long tradition of providing school reintegration in childhood cancer (see Prevatt, Heffer, & Lowe, 2000, for a review), although most programs have not been tested beyond the level of a basic program evaluation.

One recent pilot study of a school reintegration program in sickle cell disease is important and promising for several reasons (Koontz, Short, Kalinyak, & Noll, 2004). Although the sample is small ($N = 24$), students (patients) were randomized to routine care or a standardized five-step school reintegration program, notable for a highly specified protocol beginning with the initial contact with the school and concluding with a follow-up with the family and school. As predicted, the school integration program resulted in higher levels of knowledge of sickle cell disease, for children and teachers. Among the most interesting findings was that the peers of the child with sickle cell disease in the intervention arm showed significantly greater understanding and fewer misperceptions than did peers in the control group. And children in the school reintegration arm had better school attendance than did those in the control group. The potential impact of the intervention across patients, peers, and teachers is important. Interestingly, family involvement in the intervention was not achieved, a limitation noted to be important in future work integrating the school, hospital, and family.

An interesting and potentially very important illustration of a systemic intervention used with four adolescent girls with poorly controlled diabetes used multisystemic therapy (MST; Henggeler, Schoenwald, & Rowland, 2002), a flexible, family home-based intervention that involves other systems in the intervention protocol (e.g., peers, schools, communities). MST is a well-established treatment, with its roots in work with juvenile delinquency and externalizing disorders. A recent meta-analysis of MST provides strong support for its use across an impressive array of presenting problems and settings (Curtis, Ronan, & Borduin, 2004). In its first application to pediatric psychology, Ellis, Naar-King, Frey, Rowland, and Greger (2003) presented pilot data showing support for greater improvements in glycemic control for the two teens completing the

MST treatment relative to two who did not follow through with the treatment intervention. In addition to the systemic nature of MST, this approach maximizes flexibility and has proven effective with families traditionally difficult to engage in treatment. It provides an intriguing opportunity to identify pathways in the social ecology that can be identified and addressed through MST intervention strategies (Henggeler, 2003).

In conducting a systemic intervention, the locus of change might be in a system other than the family. For example, effective psychological interventions exist for procedural pain. Given the current emphasis on the development of effective and cost-efficient interventions, it is important to know whether those in the health care setting (e.g., pediatricians, nurses, social workers, and administrators) find these treatment approaches feasible and economically viable. In a procedural pain protocol that we evaluated, the Analgesia Protocol for Procedures in Oncology (Kazak, Penati, Brophy, & Himelstein, 1998), we studied the impact on staff as well as families. Initially, we described the process of introducing a family systems-oriented procedural pain treatment study and highlighted aspects of the process, including ways in which there might be understandable resistance to changing existing practices (Kazak, Blackall, Himelstein, Brophy, & Daller, 1995). In parallel with the prospective intervention study, we asked multidisciplinary staff working with children with cancer in our setting to complete questionnaires for 4 consecutive years. In this way we were able to show patterns in the acceptance and familiarity with the pain protocol and to begin to identify ways in which more effective control of patient pain could have indirect effects on staff well-being (Kazak et al., 1996).

Conceptual and Methodological Considerations
in Multiperson Intervention Research

In order to promote family intervention research in child health, difficult conceptual and methodological challenges must be addressed (Kazak, 2002a). For example, family research must measure changes not simply in one individual, but in several family members, and conceptualize how change in related individuals can be interpreted and measured. Indeed, existing measures of family functioning are insufficiently specific to pediatric illness experience and limit the ability to accurately assess change (Kazak, 2002a). As family interventions in pediatric psychology develop, it will be important for researchers to creatively address some challenges that have impeded the development in this field. These include, for example, utilizing the descriptive and explicative research on family variables to identify malleable risk and protective factors associated with disease management and to develop family assessment strategies that provide focused information to gauge the type and target of intervention.

The pragmatics of including families in research are sometimes perceived as obstacles to family intervention. There is no question that treating families requires some accommodations. One issue is flexibility in accommodating families' schedules, amplified exponentially by each family member (e.g., mother and father have different work schedules, children are busy with afterschool and evening activities). Perhaps more important is building a relationship with multiple people in the family in order to assure their participation. That is, not everyone in the family will necessarily agree on the importance of an intervention. Some families are used to delegating (e.g., "my wife handles things like that").

In pediatric conditions where many families are functioning quite competently, the way in which treatment is presented is very important. Families respond best to introductions that build on family competence and that carefully avoid invitations that make assumptions about the family's difficulties and the role of specific people in the problem. We have found, for example, in our family intervention research that families can be motivated by knowing that their efforts may help others. Such an introduction lets families enter into the intervention less defensively than if they have understood the intervention to be for families with "problems." Finally, in family treatment it is essential to include all relevant members of the family, and especially fathers, who have often been omitted in research based on convenience samples (Seagull, 2000).

Treatments for psychological difficulties are often reserved for patients and families with identified problems that warrant the attention of a consultant. While family interventions are important in these situations (Kazak, Simms, & Rourke, 2002), enhancing family functioning is also important to the prevention of problems in families with a range of levels of risk for ongoing and escalating problems.

Example of a Manualized Family Intervention

In order to illustrate a manualized family-based intervention, we present the example of the SCCIP (Kazak, Alderfer, Streisand, et al., 2004; Kazak et al., 1999).

Background

Evidence supporting the presence of PTSS in survivors and their mothers and fathers prompted us to develop an intervention to reduce PTSS. Several key findings from the literature supported the development of a multiperson intervention. First, although posttraumatic stress disorder (PTSD) itself was relatively uncommon across members of the family, PTSS were seen in all members of the family. These symptoms, such as intrusive memories about cancer and its treatment, symptoms of hyperarousal, and avoidance, are experienced within the context of the family but often not discussed among family members. By focusing on the family, the intervention could help to facilitate awareness among family members of the distress experienced by others in the family that could lead to a decrease in distress and isolation within the family. In other words, PTSS could be normalized. Indeed, in a recent study of PTSS, we found that nearly all (99%) families of survivors have at least one family member who experienced PTSS at a level to meet diagnostic criteria of the American Psychiatric Association (1994) for that symptom cluster. However, it was relatively rare for more than one person to experience PTSS at this level (or PTSD). Therefore, a family intervention would be more likely to target symptomatic family members in an efficient manner, rather than developing interventions specific to a particular family member. By extension, family members would have the opportunity to help and support one another using what they have learned from the intervention. Finally, by using proven techniques from cognitive-behavioral therapy and integrating them within a family therapy framework, it may be possible to develop an innovative and effective means of accessing more affected individuals than by working with individuals alone.

The SCCIP Protocol

SCCIP is a four-session, one-day manualized intervention to reduce PTSS in adolescent survivors of childhood cancer and their families, using a group treatment model. SCCIP was developed by a multidisciplinary team in the Division of Oncology at the Children's Hospital of Philadelphia and tested in a randomized clinical trial of 151 families (Kazak, Alderfer, Streisand, et al., 2004). Five hours of direct therapeutic contact are spread across two morning sessions that focus on cognitive-behavioral principles to reduce distress in separate groups of mothers, fathers, survivors, and siblings and two afternoon sessions that utilize family therapy approaches. Table 4.1 presents a general outline of the sessions, goals, and steps in the treatment protocol.

Table 4.1.   Outline of Sessions, Goals, and Protocol Steps in the Surviving Cancer Competently Intervention Program (SCCIP)

Session	Goals	Steps
Introduction	Introduce the program	Introduction by pediatric oncologist and psychologist, using the metaphor of cancer as a long journey
Session 1: How cancer has affected me and my family (60 min)	Establish rapport Identify group expectations Introduce background research findings	Group introductions Review research findings Identify intrusive memories Discuss how symptoms affect behavior
Session 2: Coping skills (90 min)	Introduce adversity–beliefs–consequences (ABC) model Introduce reframing Apply ABC and reframing to memories	Illustrate self-talk Present and apply ABC model Present and apply reframing
Session 3: Getting on with life: Cancer, adolescents, and families (90 min)	Understand how cancer and bothersome memories affect families and disrupt development after cancer treatment ends Identify unique ways in which cancer survival affects adolescents Facilitate connections between participants occupying analogous family, developmental, and illness roles	Presentation on cancer, families, and adolescents Multiple family discussion groups
Session 4: Pulling it all together: Family health and our future (90 min)	Review and integrate four sessions Identify how cancer affects each family Specify ways in which each family recognizes and responds to cancer-related distress Formulate and practice ways of "putting cancer in its place"	Summary of first three sessions and plans for this session Intrafamily discussion of four questions (recognizing distress, responding to distress, putting illness in its place, next steps for family) Large group discussion: how to put what was learned into action for the ongoing growth and development

The introduction to the SCCIP intervention day is provided jointly by a psychologist and an oncologist, in order to emphasize the integration of health and well-being and the concern for the long-term health of cancer survivors. In Session 1 ("How Cancer Has Affected Me and My Family"), traumatic memories of cancer are identified in group formats that are designed with attention to enhancing the cohesiveness and supportiveness of the group. The protocols for the mother and father groups are identical. For the teen groups (survivors, siblings), the formats are similar but with utilization of age-appropriate examples and prompts, including an icebreaker and use of cartoons.

In presenting and working with the cognitive-behavioral approaches used in Session 2 ("Coping Skills"), interventionist adherence and competence ratings include consideration of their success in engaging in and encouraging interactions among group members. As illustrated in table 4.2, subsequent to introducing the concept of self-talk and the adversity–beliefs–consequences (ABC) model generally, cancer-specific examples are used. Again, interaction among the group members is expected, and the therapist helps participants to apply what they have learned to their family as well as to themselves individually, in anticipation of the afternoon family therapy sessions.

Session 3 ("Getting on With Life: Cancer, Adolescents, and Families") uses an adaptation of multiple family discussion groups (MFDGs) in order to facilitate an understanding of how beliefs about cancer today continue to impact members of the family. MFDGs are established interventions that have been used in severe psychiatric disorders (McFarlane, 2002) and chronic child and adult illnesses (Gonzalez, Steinglass, & Reiss, 1989; Ostroff & Steinglass, 1996; Satin et al., 1989; Steinglass, 1998; Steinglass, Gonzales, Dosovitz, & Reiss, 1982; Wamboldt & Levin, 1995). MFDGs provide for discussion and observation of family members as they discuss the impact of illness on the family. The protocol stipulates that people in each role (survivor, mother, father, sibling) sequentially have a small group discussion for 10 minutes about "how their beliefs about cancer affect their family today." Then, the observers (other family members) discuss what they heard. Thus, a small group of mothers has the first discussion, followed by a discussion of what the observers (fathers, siblings, survivors) heard. (See figure 4.2 for an illustration and tables 4.3 and 4.4 for excerpts from the treatment manual for Session 3.) This is followed by discussion of survivors, siblings, and fathers, including the observer discussion after each. MFDGs are a powerful technique because people hear both their family

Table 4.2.   Using the ABC Model in Groups of Mothers and Groups of Fathers

	Steps
Prior steps in the session	Presentation and examples of self-talk Presentation of ABC model (general example)

ABC model
(cancer example);
uses flipcharts
	Now we will apply this model to some current situations that may trigger bothersome memories of your child's cancer. Most of you return to clinic for follow-up visits. This remains a major adversity.
	    A. Adversity: The "A" would be returning to clinic for follow-up visits, which triggers bothersome memories of cancer and its treatment.
	    B. Beliefs: The "B" would be the thoughts or beliefs that you had about the visit and about the cancer generally. Perhaps you thought to yourself, "What if he or she has relapsed or recurred. What if they find a new problem? Maybe his or her existing difficulties will be worse. I am not sure if my child will ever have a normal life."
	    C. Emotional Consequences: The "C" would be the fear and anxiety that you feel days or weeks before the clinic visit. What you said to yourself about returning to clinic, in other words, your beliefs, increased the fear and anxiety.
	Your thoughts about returning to clinic influenced how you felt. B influences C. Thoughts influence feelings. Your beliefs about what might happen at a follow-up visit and the resulting fear and anxiety contribute to how bothersome your memories are to you, now and in the future. Before we move on, are there any questions?
	Now, we would like you to focus on the bothersome memories that you chose in the first session. Please refer to your ABC worksheets. You are going to apply the ABC model to your own bothersome memories. . . .

Reframing beliefs; uses flipcharts and handouts	*Now we are going to help you look at adversities or problems in a new way using a tool called reframing beliefs. Reframing means changing the way you look at things. This tool will help you to identify and change unhelpful beliefs or thoughts. Unhelpful beliefs and thoughts increase negative feelings, such as fear, anxiety, and anger. Identifying unhelpful beliefs, and reframing them, will help you to change the intensity of your feelings.* *Changing B can change C. Changing your thoughts can change your feelings.* *The change, however, will not be immediate. You must practice reframing beliefs and thoughts. Over time, you may feel better.* *(Continued)*

Table 4.2. *(Continued)*

Steps
Reframing beliefs has three parts: accept the uncontrollable, focus on the controllable, and use the positive. *1. Accept the uncontrollable: Accept the uncontrollable means accepting that which you cannot change.* *2. Focus on the controllable: Focus on the controllable means focus on that which you can change.* *3. Use the positive: There are two ways to use the positive. First, identify the realistically positive aspects of a situation. Next, acknowledge your own competence or ability to deal with a situation. All of these suggestions need to be realistic for you and your family at this point in time.* *Changing B through reframing beliefs can change C.* *Changing your thoughts can change your feelings.*

Note. Reprinted from Session 2 in *Surviving Cancer Competently Intervention Program Manual*, by A. Kazak (unpublished).

member and others in comparable roles from other families talk about the impact of cancer on the family. Typically, families indicate that they have not had discussions like this before. Session 4 brings family members together, with the task of answering four questions related to their beliefs about cancer and their future (table 4.5).

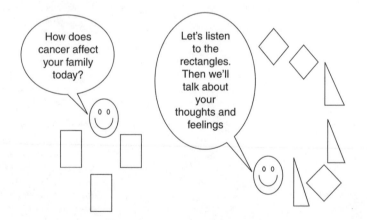

Figure 4.2　Illustration of multiple family discussion groups. The small group of rectangles represents family members (e.g., mothers) having a discussion, and the triangles and diamonds represent other family members listening. After this conversation ends, the larger group of other family members closes its circle to have a discussion about what its members heard the mothers say. The mothers open up their circle and listen to this conversation. The procedure repeats for groups of survivors, siblings, and fathers.

Table 4.3. Family Discussion of Impact of Cancer Survival on the Family

	Steps
Prior steps in the session	Review format of Sessions 3 and 4 (multiple family discussion groups and session with one's own family) Introduce impact of cancer survival on families
Discussion of impact of cancer survival on families; uses cartoons	(Facilitate a discussion, using an easel and paper for notes. Begin with the cartoon showing the family with multiple bubbles illustrating the possible impact of cancer on family life as a prompt for discussions. Introduce the cartoon.) *Here is a family of a childhood cancer survivor. There is a lot going on in their lives. Let's start our discussion of how cancer affects families by talking about how cancer has affected this family. How has cancer affected this family? What is this family struggling with?* (Transition to soliciting participants' ideas related to the general question: How does cancer affect families? Keep the discussion moving. Be sure to cover the points mentioned, if participants do not raise them. Sample prompt questions are included. General prompt: *How does cancer change how families work?*) *Cancer affects the entire family. During the treatment phase, cancer played a central role in your lives. You had to balance jobs, family life, and treatment—you may not have had much time together. You endured the stress of seeing your child uncomfortable. You always worried about what was ahead. Family and child development was disrupted. Your other children may have felt left out. You figured out ways to "get back on track."* (General prompt: *How about kids? How does cancer affect how kids grow up?*) *You had many painful procedures. You missed school and other activities with your family and friends. You were scared or knew that your parents felt upset. Siblings felt cut off from the family and often felt that they did not know what was going on. Cancer can be a roadblock to independence. You may feel different because cancer has changed you. You have more responsibility, including having to decide what to tell people about cancer. Cancer can make some decisions more difficult (e.g., dating, jobs, health issues).* (General prompt: *What do families expect when treatment ends?*) *When treatment ended, you may have been told that you can resume a "normal" life. The map for how to resume life after cancer is not well charted. Beliefs that you found helpful during treatment may not be*

(Continued)

Table 4.3. (*Continued*)

	Steps
	helpful any longer. It's hard to put the illness aside and move on. Worries about the future continue. (General Prompt: *How do you talk about cancer?*) *You may struggle with how to talk about your experiences. You might wonder whether other family members have similar thoughts or beliefs. Sometimes you may feel preoccupied or alone when you remember cancer. You may assume that your experiences and thoughts are different from other people's. Talking can reduce isolation and increase feelings of connectedness.*

Note. Reprinted from Session 3 in *Surviving Cancer Competently Intervention Program Manual,* by A. Kazak (unpublished).

Table 4.4. Family Discussion of Impact of Cancer Survival on the Family

	Steps
Prior steps	Discussion of impact of cancer survival on families
First MFDG	*Let's start by having the mothers pull their chairs into a small circle. Everyone else, please form a larger circle around this inner group.* Interventionist A: With each person seated: *We are going to divide our time into four discussion sessions. In the first session, the mothers will sit in a circle with me. The mothers will talk for 10 minutes about how cancer affects them today. Everyone else will be observers and then have a 10-minute discussion about what they heard the mothers say. We will repeat this for teens, siblings, and then for fathers.* Interventionist A: *We would like you to talk with each other as if your families were not here. This may seem difficult, or unnatural, but let's give it a try.* Interventionist B reinforces this with observers: *We are going to listen during this part. But while we listen, it's important to pay attention to our own thoughts and reactions for discussion later.* Interventionist A: *Now, we'd like you to discuss this question: How do your beliefs about cancer affect your family today? That is, how do the beliefs that you identified this morning impact your family?* (We have found that this more focused question is important. Whereas more general questions will elicit valuable discussion, this focused question provides a tight link with the morning session. As a short discussion, the interventionist should keep the group as focused as possible. If the group has difficulty (*Continued*)

Table 4.4. (*Continued*)

	Steps
	getting started, the leader can refer them to the cards that they chose as bothersome memories, or prompt them. They should be encouraged to talk with one another, not to the interventionist). After 10 minutes: *Thank you. A number of important ideas and feelings have come up here. Now let's hear what the observers have to say.* (Chairs are moved as in figure 4.1, from the multiple family group discussion format.)
Observer discussion	Interventionist B with observers: *What came to mind as you listened to the mothers? How do their beliefs affect how your family acts? How are their ideas similar or different from what you believe? You may have had a reaction to what your family member said, or to the group of mothers as a whole. We would like the observers to talk as a group about the general messages that you heard.* (This is a 10-minute discussion between the group members within each subgroup, encouraging discussion of similar and contrasting views. Facilitators should try not to feel constrained by the short amount of time allotted, but rather facilitate and probe as indicated clinically. Families should be increasingly aware of differing perspectives within families and that they as a group must take these differing viewpoints and feelings into account. The co-leaders should discourage cross-group discussion because they will interfere with the structural intervention intended by organizing members along illness-role lines rather than by families. Subgroup participants should be encouraged to talk among themselves, rather than to the leaders. Sometimes this can be facilitated with questions such as, "Has anyone else had a similar or different reaction?" or "What are other people's thoughts about what _____ had to say?"
Next steps	This repeats for small group discussions by survivors, siblings, and fathers.

Note. Reprinted from Session 3 in *Surviving Cancer Competently Intervention Program Manual,* by A. Kazak (unpublished).

Our approach to writing the manual was to be as specific as possible in terms of offering scripted text. In training interventionists (including nurses, nurse practitioners, social workers, and trainees as well as psychologists), we cover basic family therapy skills in order to allow the interventionists to put their conversations with families into their own words, while retaining treatment fidelity. For example, encouraging interactions among the members of groups

Table 4.5. Consolidating Learning From the SCCIP Intervention and Looking to the Future

	Steps
Prior steps	Reorganize families and chairs (one large group)
Review of prior sessions; present format for Session 4	*Throughout this program we have talked about how cancer impacts teenagers, siblings, parents, and families. In the first session each of you identified three bothersome memories. Then you applied the ABC reframing model to these bothersome memories. With practice, this tool can help reduce the impact of these memories. In the last session, family members talked about their current beliefs about cancer and how their thoughts and beliefs affect families. You talked with members of other families. You also had the chance to sit back and listen to your family, and others, describe the ways in which cancer affects them today. You may have heard ways in which people in the same family see things very differently. These different perspectives influence how your family works.* *In this session we will pull all the work that you have done together. Our goal is to have you think through what your "take home" message will be. How do you think your family will change as a result of this experience? How will your family use what you've learned today? Who will take the lead in making this a part of your lives at home?* *You will be with your family and asked to discuss four questions that relate to how cancer affects you today. For each, your family will be asked to write a few phrases or sentences on a worksheet. At the end of the session, you will share what your family has done with the group. Please choose a member of your family to speak for your family to the larger group.*
Four questions for the future	(One interventionist reads the four questions, which are passed out to families on worksheets. The other interventionists sit with the families when the questions are read and discussed. Their tasks are to observe, clarify the questions, expand discussion when families are "stuck," or focus the discussion if appears unfocused.) *Please move your chairs so that you are sitting with your family. Your family will be asked four questions. Please listen to each question. Then discuss your typical response. When you have one or two answers that fit your family, please write them on the worksheet. Don't worry if you haven't fully discussed the questions. We expect that you will want to continue talking about these questions after you leave.* *The first two questions are grouped together. The first is: How do we know when our beliefs about cancer are*

(Continued)

Table 4.5.   (Continued)

	Steps
	causing distress in our family today? The second question is: How do we respond to each other's distress? Please discuss your responses. Then write your family responses on the worksheet, where it says "Beliefs about cancer cause distress in our family today by . . ." and "We respond to each other's distress by . . ."
Next steps	Large group discussion with sharing of work from families with one another.
	Completion of program evaluation questionnaire.

Note. Reprinted from Session 4 in *Surviving Cancer Competently Intervention Program Manual,* by A. Kazak (unpublished).

(whether they are mothers, fathers, etc., or family groups) is necessary in order to score at the highest level of competence in our treatment fidelity approach. Role-playing activities during training include family therapy techniques such as joining (Kazak et al., 2002) and using the ARCH (acceptance, respect, curiosity, honesty) of therapy, as described by Micucci (1998).

Helpful Hints

Given the diverse range of interventions covered in this chapter, it is difficult to succinctly capture hints for conducting family interventions in the same manner as those provided for individual therapies (see chapter 3). However, some general guidelines can be offered that help orient pediatric psychologists toward working with families.

1. *Identify who is in the family.* The stereotype of "family" as consisting of a two-parent heterosexual unit with biological children from that marriage has persisted despite ample evidence for the diversity of family structures. Working with families necessitates basic consideration of who is in the family, from the family's perspective (Kazak, 2003a).

2. *Realize that families are greater than the sum of their parts.* Clinical work with multiple members of the family does not necessarily represent a family systems approach. Across family theories and family therapy models are assumptions of complex interactions that define a system that is broader and different from the sum of any of its parts.

3. *Attain skills for conducting multiperson interventions.* In most pediatric psychology programs and internships, relatively little attention is given to specific training in family therapy approaches. Competent work with families requires coursework and hands-on supervised work in the complexities of family assessment and therapy (Kazak, 2003b).

4. *Embrace the competence of families in pediatric health care.* Many of the assumptions underlying traditional models of psychotherapy are ill-suited to families of pediatric patients. Most families are relatively highly functioning and are learning to adjust and live with diseases and treatments that challenge and change their existing family lives. Interventions with families should be appropriately matched to the level of distress and needs expressed.

III COMMON TOPICS IN PEDIATRIC PSYCHOLOGY INTERVENTION

5 Pain

Pediatric psychologists have contributed consistently and broadly to the systematic assessment and treatment of pain in infants, children, and adolescents. Increasing attention over the last decade to the issue of pain in the medical management of children has resulted in additional opportunities for the utilization of pain management protocols in pediatric settings. In the *Journal of Pediatric Psychology* (*JPP*) Empirically Supported Treatments Series, four separate articles reviewed the existing literature on pediatric pain. The four areas were recurrent pediatric headache (Holden, Deichmann, & Levy, 1999), recurrent abdominal pain (RAP; Janicke & Finney, 1999), procedure-related pain (Powers, 1999), and disease-related pain (Walco, Sterling, Conte, & Engel, 1999). Since the publication of the *JPP* Empirically Supported Treatments Series articles on pain, there have been a few psychosocial treatment studies on disease-related pain, several treatment studies on headache and RAP, and a fairly large number on procedure-related pain.

In this chapter, we introduce the different pain topics, review the findings of the *JPP* Empirically Supported Treatments Series paper on that topic, and provide an update on intervention studies. We review the use of biofeedback when discussing headaches because it is commonly used in the treatment of pain secondary to headaches. The protocol described can be easily adapted for both RAP and disease-related pain. Working with parents is emphasized in the clinical section on RAP. The parent component described in the clinical section on RAP is pertinent to many children with headaches and can be easily adapted for these children. Under procedure-related pain, we describe the behavioral treatment protocols used in the most recent studies on this topic. Detailed descriptions of behavioral treatments for many different types of procedure-related pain (e.g., injections, IVs, etc.) are also readily available to pediatric psychologists elsewhere (e.g., Chen, Joseph, & Zeltzer, 2000). Consequently, our discussion of clinical approaches for procedure-related pain is limited to a protocol for parents of very young children and a self-control procedure for school-age children. Finally, under disease-related pain, we review some clinical considerations specific to pain that presents secondary to disease states.

Pediatric Recurrent Headache

Headaches are relatively common presenting problems for pediatricians, can have a variety of etiologies, and represent a range of diagnostic entities, most commonly migraine and tension headaches. Of particular concern are recurrent headaches in which the chronic nature of headache interferes with the child's daily functioning. About 50% of children report experiencing headaches at least monthly (Cady, Farmer, Griesemer, & Sable, 1996). Holden and associates identified 31 intervention studies related to recurrent headaches in their review article (Holden et al., 1999). Interventions that utilize relaxation or variants of relaxation procedures, such as self-hypnosis and guided imagery, are well-established interventions for pediatric recurrent headache. A second group of interventions were those that utilized biofeedback for pediatric headache. This treatment approach was also viewed as probably effective based on the literature reviewed and can be recommended as a helpful treatment for pediatric recurrent headache. The findings on biofeedback, however, are typically confounded by the fact that relaxation training is included in the biofeedback protocol.

Intervention Studies of Pediatric Headache Published Since 1999

An interesting update to the literature on cognitive-behavioral treatments for headaches was conducted in Germany, comparing a therapist-administered, eight-session group cognitive-behavioral intervention (TG; $N = 29$) with a self-help format (SH; $N = 27$) and a wait-list control group ($N = 19$; Kroener-Herwig & Denecke, 2002). The group sessions lasted 90 minutes and included education about headache causes and etiology, the effects of stress on headaches and how to cope with stress, the role of negative cognitions in pain and stress, progressive relaxation techniques, imagery and distraction, self-assertion, problem solving, and application of these approaches to prevent and treat headaches. The SH group received the same content but in a self-help format. The SH children were contacted by phone each week. The therapist checked on their progress using the self-help manual and any problems the children encountered. The two active treatments were superior to the wait-list control group in reducing the frequency and intensity of headaches. By the end of treatment, about half of the children in the treatment group demonstrated clinically relevant headache improvement. At 6-month follow-up, 76% of the TG group and 68% of the SH group reported significant improvement in their headaches. The two treatment groups did not differ in terms of outcomes (headache intensity, duration, and frequency), although effect sizes were noted to be larger for the TG group than for the SH group, supportive of the earlier findings of P. J. McGrath et al. (1992) in showing that self-help materials are useful although somewhat less efficacious than therapist-guided intervention.

An innovative and potentially cost-effective approach to pediatric headache was described by Andrasik et al. (2003), using an 8-week group intervention. The patients were seen in small group sessions of three to five children lasting for 30 minutes. The eight-session group intervention was similar to the Kroener-Herwig and Denecke (2002) group format. It included coping skills to apply to prevent and reduce headache pain, progressive muscle relaxation, and audiotapes to promote practice between sessions. Children were asked to practice daily during the 8-week group treatment and twice weekly at the conclusion of treatment designed by a psychologist but led by a neurologist. Thirty-seven patients participated in this uncontrolled study, with the authors indicating improvements in number of headache days as well as emotional distress. Almost 80% of the children reported a greater than 50% reduction in headache days from baseline to 12-month follow-up which was maintained at 1-year follow-up (Andrasik et al., 2003). Biofeedback involves the electronic monitoring, measurement, and display of physiological processes that are normally beyond conscious awareness but that, when observed, can come under voluntary control. Instrumentation is used to monitor the physiological effects of relaxation and facilitate the learning of relaxation skills by providing visual or audio feedback about actual changes in otherwise invisible bodily processes. The feedback is usually given via an audio or a visual display. For children, displays are usually gamelike, utilizing graphics and audio feedback.

Holroyd et al. (1984) suggest that there are two mechanisms by which biofeedback results in symptom improvement. First, some individuals learn to control a physiologic response, such as muscle tension, via biofeedback training and then use that control, as needed, to reduce symptoms, such as tension headaches. Second, in most cases, cognitive change is a more likely result of biofeedback training. That is, individuals perceive that they are successful in controlling a physiologic response, and this perception improves their overall feeling of self-efficacy. An enhanced feeling of self-efficacy leads to more successful coping efforts, lower stress, and improved symptoms.

Further support for biofeedback in the treatment of pediatric migraine is seen in three studies, each with a relatively small sample but with consistent evidence for the effectiveness of biofeedback, as well as supporting its application in practice. In one study, 36 patients were randomly assigned to hand-warming thermal biofeedback plus stress management techniques, hand-cooling thermal biofeedback plus stress management, or an attention or wait-list control condition (Scharff, Marcus, & Masek, 2002). The hand-warming biofeedback group received four 1-hour sessions in a 6-week period that combined cognitive-behavioral stress management training with 30 minutes of thermal biofeedback training. The stress management procedure included thought stopping, positive self-statements, and identification of stressful situations and stressful thinking. Imagery of warm places plus deep breathing was used to increase peripheral finger temperature. Each biofeedback session consisted of 4 minutes of habitation, 20 minutes of hand-warming (or hand-cooling) exercises with feedback, and 6 minutes of return to baseline without feedback. Children in both biofeedback groups improved, suggesting there are nonspecific effects associated with biofeedback treatment. However, hand warming was associated with greater improvement than was hand cooling. The sample size and the mixed intervention (biofeedback and stress management) limit the conclusions that can be drawn.

In another study of 20 children with migraine headache, biofeedback was used to assess their ability to learn and use techniques for changing peripheral body temperature (PBT) using a 1-hour relaxation intervention provided within a multidisciplinary headache clinic (Powers et al., 2001). All patients also received pharmacologic treatment. The relaxation procedure was audiotaped, and the children were asked to practice at least three times per week for 2 weeks at the onset of a headache. Follow-up data were collected at the first or second follow-up medical visit, which occurred over about a 6-month period. The data suggest that children can be taught to use biofeedback techniques to increase PBT within a 1-hour session and that the successful mastery of these techniques resulted in somewhat less headache discomfort and better functionality. Specifically, average headache frequency reduced from about 13 to 10 days per month, and average headache duration decreased from about 7 to 5 hours.

Arndorfer and Allen (2001) used a similar thermal biofeedback protocol with five children, 8 to 14 years of age, with tension, rather than migraine, headaches. The children were seen for four weekly sessions of thermal biofeedback and two follow-up sessions. Each session consisted of 10 minutes of habitation and 10 minutes of hand-warming, imagery practice. Feedback regarding the physiologic results of the imagery procedure was given to the child during a 5-minute rest period. The last 10 minutes consisted of a feedback session in which the physiologic data was displayed to the child. Children were instructed to practice the imagery procedure at home twice per day for 10 minutes each. All patients demonstrated clinically significant reductions in one or more headache parameters, and four of five were headache-free at 6 months.

Finally, a pain management package including biofeedback, which was administered by a master's level clinician without specific training in biofeedback, was tested in a multiple-baseline-design study of pediatric headache (Allen, Elliott, & Arndorfer, 2002). The intervention was delivered in a primary care setting to seven children. They received five sessions of thermal biofeedback, with each session lasting 10 to 15 minutes. Inexpensive alcohol thermometers were given to each child, and they were instructed to practice the hand-warming procedure at least once per day at home and record their practice results. Later sessions were used to promote generalization, and children were instructed to use the procedure at the first sign of headache onset. Improvements in one or more headache parameters (i.e., intensity, duration, and frequency) were found for six of the seven patients. The one child who did not improve had daily continuous headaches that are often found to be nonresponsive to medical and psychological treatments.

In summary, intervention studies published subsequent to *JPP*'s Empirically Supported Treatments Series paper on pediatric recurrent headache support the conclusions of Holden et al. (1999). In the absence of further randomized clinical trials in this field, there are no changes to Holden et al.'s earlier conclusions. Of note is the increasing emphasis in the studies on brief, easy-to-administer, cost-effective treatments for headache.

Using Biofeedback for Headache in Clinical Practice

Below we outline a general approach for the use of biofeedback in the treatment of pediatric headache. These procedures should be used in the context of an overall pain management protocol such as the one described by Allen and Mathews (1998). Two parameters considered correlates of tension and migraine headaches are most commonly used in biofeedback training with children and adolescents. The first is electromyographic (EMG) activity, electrical discharge in the muscle fibers, a correlate of skeletal muscle tension. EMG activity is typically measured by placement of an electrode on the forehead in the treatment of tension headaches. The second, skin temperature, a correlate of vasomotor control mechanisms, is typically measured peripherally via a finger in the treatment of migraine headache. The rationale provided to patients is that blood vessel constriction followed by dilation is responsible for migraine pain. Monitoring finger temperature is described as an indirect way of measuring blood flow, which in turn is related to stress and migraine headaches. Developing the ability to dilate blood vessels is presumed to produce a stabilizing effect on the peripheral vasculature system. In more recent conceptualizations of headache, the pathophysiology of both migraine and tension headaches is believed to be an overreactive vasomotor system, and both types of headaches are believed to involve vascular and skeletal muscle factors (Viswanathan, Bridges, Whitehouse, & Newton, 1998). Therefore, no matter what type of headache is being treated, either tension or migraine, both EMG and finger temperature are often monitored and feedback given on one or both parameters, at least partially because children may be more reactive and better able to achieve physiologic change in one parameter than the other.

A typical headache treatment protocol is 8 to 12 sessions over a 3- to 4-month period. A baseline evaluation is conducted first to assess the physiologic parameters of interest. The child is asked to sit quietly in a room without moving too much (to avoid movement artifact) for a 5-minute period to assess resting levels of EMG frontalis activity and peripheral finger temperature. Second, a very common assessment procedure is to present some sort of stressor, such as difficult math problems or a stressful interpersonal situation, to see any changes in physiologic response. For clinical purposes, it is also usually best to pick a stressor that is related to the child's headaches, such as having a test in school the next day or having a fight with a sibling.

After the baseline session, the child is taught a relaxation procedure (see chapter 3). The child's physiologic responses are monitored while he or she is relaxing. In subsequent biofeedback training sessions, a brief habituation period is followed by a baseline period of 5 to 8 minutes. Baseline is followed by periods of relaxation with and without feedback in 5-minute blocks for up to 20 minutes. Depending on the protocol, a return to baseline may follow each period of relaxation or feedback.

In the feedback trial, the child is given immediate access to his or her physiologic readings (feedback). In the most typical scenario, while a child is relaxing, a visual cue or audio signal is provided to the child. The child is typically instructed to try to relax and then to look toward the screen occasionally or listen to the tone to determine the efficacy of the relaxing. If the feedback indicates the child is not relaxing well, then that is the signal to try other approaches to relaxation. For example, if a child is using a meditative breathing technique, shifting to imagery-based relaxation might be a way to improve the physiologic responses. In turn, the feedback from the TV screen or the audio signal tells the child if the shift in relaxation has helped improve the physiologic response.

Some children find the feedback very helpful and enjoyable and like to spend a good deal of the session using feedback trials to improve their skills. Others find that either the audio or visual signal is a distraction from relaxation and does not enhance their ability to relax. Consequently, they say they would rather just relax and have their trial monitored than receive feedback during the trial. Achieving a goal set by the therapist, such as reducing frontalis EMG by 1 microvolt, is often intrinsically reinforcing. Although children may be willing to work for the sounding of an audio signal from the biofeedback equipment, it is also useful to provide extrinsic reinforcement, such as being allowed to play computer games as a reward for attaining a specific goal. Some children and adolescents become upset during a feedback trial if they are unable to produce results (e.g., a lowering of the EMG frontalis level). In most of these cases, frustration causes a significant rise in muscle tension or drop in finger temperature. Thus, the physical effects of the stress response are demonstrated quite readily to the child, and the ensuing expectations for achievement become a topic for discussion and work in sessions.

After each one of these trials—the baseline trial, the stressor trial, and the monitored relaxation trial—the data are saved and displayed in some user-friendly fashion. It is then helpful for the clinician to review the results of these sessions with the child to highlight the relationship between stress and physiologic responses or relaxation and physiologic response.

One approach is to conduct treatment until the symptom abates. Those who advocate this approach want to achieve a treatment effect. Others maintain that it is the patient's ability to control a physiologic response that is critical, and consequently that treatment should continue until a specified physiologic outcome is achieved, such as the ability to lower EMG 2 microvolts or raise finger temperature to 95 degrees—even if symptoms have already been eliminated.

As with relaxation training, the cognitive and attentional demands of the treatment make biofeedback best suited for children 7 years and older. They must also be able to maintain attention and concentrate on their bodily sensations for an extended time. Children need to be able to understand the rationale of using biofeedback equipment for their problem. It is important to describe to the child just what happens in biofeedback and to allay any apprehension the child has about the equipment. Clear, developmentally appropriate, and repeated explanations of the procedures and devices should be provided to both children and parents. Technical terms such as conductance, electrodes, and so forth, should be avoided. Make sure the child understands that the wires running to the forehead will not cause an electric shock.

Parents should be included in sessions whenever possible so they can encourage the child's practice at home. In addition, the consequences of having a headache, such as social reinforcement by parents or avoidance of negative circumstances (e.g., school, peers), should be examined to ensure these factors are not maintaining the headaches. No matter what factors are related to the child's headaches, children should be encouraged to maintain their normal activities or resume their activities as soon as possible. In addition, parents should encourage the child to try to handle the headache by using their relaxation procedures and praise the child when he or she manages a headache well.

Recurrent Abdominal Pain

RAP is a complex pediatric problem at the interface of psychological and physiological symptomatology. Factors both psychological, such as stress and somatization disorders, and physiological, such as lactose intolerance and gut motility, have been suggested as causes. With highest incidence in the elementary school years, about 10% to 15% of this age group may have RAP and seek guidance from pediatricians and psychologists regarding stomach pain and related gastrointestinal symptoms with no organic etiology identifiable (Janicke & Finney, 1999). RAP pain is paroxysmal, occurs three or more times over a 3-month period, and interrupts normal activities.

The conceptualization of RAP as a condition involving both psychological and physiological factors can be confusing to patients and parents. Health care providers often have difficulty knowing how best to explain RAP and treat these symptoms, which can result in functional impairment, later psychological difficulties, and increasing health care utilization and cost. A reassuring, clear, and non-blaming explanation for RAP is important and often sufficient to help patients and parents address concerns that may be causing or exacerbating the pain. Providing an accurate explanation is typically the first line of intervention that should not be overlooked in terms of its potential positive impact (Banez & Cunningham, 2003).

Due to the complexity of RAP, psychological intervention is often critically important to help children and families reduce the distress experienced. Janicke and Finney (1999) reviewed nine intervention studies in this area, grouping them into three categories of intervention: operant procedures, fiber treatments, and cognitive-behavioral approaches. Based on the literature at that time, it was concluded that fiber treatments were promising interventions. Sufficient evidence was presented for cognitive-behavioral interventions to be recognized as having a probably efficacious rating due largely to the lack of intervention studies across research groups.

Intervention Studies for Pediatric RAP Published Since 1999

Only three intervention studies have been reported subsequent to the review by Janicke and Finney (1999). There is no additional strong empirical support for specific psychological interventions in this important area of work, although the results of one randomized controlled trial are supportive of a cognitive-behavioral and family intervention for RAP (Robins, Smith, Glutting, & Bishop, in press). Sixty-nine children with RAP were randomized into standard medical care ($N = 29$) or standard medical care plus a cognitive-behavioral family intervention ($N = 40$). Standard medical care included office visits, education, dietary recommendations, and possible medication or supplements to increase fiber and reduce stomach acidity and motility. In the cognitive-behavioral family intervention group, parents and children learned about recurrent stomach pain and cognitive-behavioral strategies for active pain management. Parents received coaching on ways of enhancing their child's coping with pain (Robins et al., in press). The intervention was conducted over five bimonthly sessions. In addition to data collected 3 months after the intervention data, a follow-up data point was included 6–12 months after study entry. The results show that both groups improved in child- and parent-reported pain and overall functioning. However, the group receiving the psychological intervention showed greater improvement in pain, a finding that persisted over 1 year. There was also significant evidence for better school attendance in this treatment arm (Robins et al., in press). This paper is supportive of the earlier reports of cognitive-behavioral family intervention by Sanders and colleagues (Sanders et al., 1989; Sanders, Shepherd, Cleghorn, & Woolford, 1994). Although the interventions are not identical, their similar conceptual basis and methodologies help to move this work in the direction of an efficacious treatment for RAP.

In a study that is consistent with prior research, Humphreys and Gevirtz (2000) randomly assigned children with RAP (*N* = 64) to four treatment arms: fiber-only comparison group; fiber and biofeedback; fiber, biofeedback, and cognitive-behavioral intervention; and fiber, biofeedback, cognitive-behavioral intervention, and parent support. The cognitive-behavioral protocol was adapted from that used by Sanders et al. (1994) in prior studies and began with an explanation of RAP, pain, and pain-related behavior. Relaxation training, coping statements, distraction techniques, and self-management strategies were the focus of treatment. Thermal biofeedback was used to monitor increases in finger temperature that occurred secondary to use of relaxation and self-control strategies. Identification of high-risk situations and relapse prevention procedures were also taught. Finally, to ensure that the children understood the cognitive component of training, they were asked to teach the cognitive skills to the interventionist and then to the parents. All groups were noted to show symptomatic improvement. The small sample and complex study design make it difficult to draw conclusions supportive of specific intervention approaches.

Anbar (2001) taught self-hypnosis to five pediatric RAP patients and reported resolution of RAP symptoms within 3 weeks for four of the patients. The lack of a controlled design and absence of clear inclusion criteria limit any conclusions from this report and add minimally to the conclusions of Janicke and Finney (1999).

Using Cognitive-Behavioral Therapy in Clinical Practice for RAP

Cognitive-behavioral therapy (CBT) treatment protocols are probably efficacious for the management of pain associated with RAP. These protocols typically consist of a child self-management component and a parent component. The child self-management component uses techniques found to treat both headaches and disease-related pain. These techniques include relaxation training, positive imagery, coping self-statements, and distraction. These approaches are discussed elsewhere in this volume (chapter 3) and are not repeated here.

RAP protocols almost always use verbal instructions, written guidelines for parents and children, in-session modeling of the techniques, in-session practice of the techniques, parent instruction in coaching and reinforcing the child's use of the techniques, homework, practice assignments, and reinforcement (Sanders et al., 1994). The CBT protocol described by Sanders et al. (1994) includes an imagery technique in which the child is asked to imagine a favorite cartoon character "eating" the pain away. The protocol includes a final session in relapse prevention in which children are presented with a personalized high-risk situation, such as taking a big test in school, and asked to problem-solve around strategies they would implement to prevent the onset of pain and also how to manage pain at the first sign of its occurrence.

Working collaboratively with parents is essential. A critical component of RAP protocols are approaches provided to parents to help them understand and systematically address behavioral signs of their child's pain (e.g., moaning, verbal complaints, holding or rubbing the area of pain, etc.), not just the child's subjective experience of pain. Pain treatment programs spend a significant portion of time helping parents discriminate between pain behaviors that are not urgent and complaints of acute symptoms that require immediate attention (e.g., a new pattern of symptoms suggesting a new illness other than RAP; Sanders et al., 1994). In an acute pain situation, attention to the child's pain complaints and pain behavior is appropriate parenting. If the child is ill or uncomfortable, parents should respond to try to help their child. This is different from circumstances in which acute pain becomes frequent recurring pain, such as in the case of RAP and headaches. In these instances, parents are coached to understand how frequent attention to the pain behaviors may result in inadvertent reinforcement of "pain behavior" rather than "well behavior." As an example, parents may note that if their child lies down or is inactive, then pain improves. Although this may be true, long periods of inactivity do not eventually resolve the child's pain and are more likely to have negative effects on the child's overall social-emotional functioning (Dahlquist & Switkin, 2003).

The importance of encouraging well behavior and coping behavior is also stressed. Parents may attend more to the child when he or she is in pain, comforting them and soothing them, and then be relieved when the child is no longer in pain and does not "bother them" when he or she is feeling well, thus ignoring well behavior. Or parents may feel closer to their child when attending to their child's pain or use this time spent with their child to avoid a stressful circumstance, such as work or marital conflict (Walker, 1999). Particularly in cases where the child and the family feel frustrated with progress in understanding and treating the child's pain, a sense of "us" (family) against "them" (health care team) can develop (P. J. McGrath & Feldman, 1986).

Other examples in which children are potentially rewarded for pain behavior are seen in instances in which children receive gifts from family members when they are sick or in pain. Teachers and classmates may also pay more attention to the child with a painful medical condition. Children may escape from chores or schoolwork by being in pain or terminate stressful family interactions with pain complaints (Dahlquist & Switkin, 2003).

Children who are not functioning optimally—for example, have peer relationship issues, school problems, or perceive themselves to be incompetent in some fashion—may be more at risk to restrict activities, withdraw, and seek attention in response to pain (Walker, 1999). This may be particularly true for children who set high internal standards for academic performance, are in a highly competitive academic or extracurricular situation, or are in highly stressful home situations (Walker, 1999). In some protocols, parents are first asked to monitor their discussions of pain with their child (Finney, Lemanek, Cataldo, Katz, & Fuqua, 1989). This can facilitate awareness of the extent to which pain has become the focus of interaction at home. Once parents understand the rationale for minimizing attention to their child's behavior, they are urged to prompt children to engage in coping behaviors, to substitute other behaviors, or to use distraction when their child complains of pain. Simultaneously, situations in which parents may ignore nonverbal expression of pain (e.g., grimacing, moaning), model coping behavior, and avoid modeling sick role behaviors are illustrated (Sanders et al., 1994). In this way, parents are coached to attend to well behavior and to offer the child reinforcement for these other behaviors.

Procedure-Related Pain

Invasive and potentially painful procedures are an essential part of pediatric health care. Procedures include injections ("shots") that are relatively common in pediatric practice, generally short in duration, and with short-term acute pain and distress on the child's part. Alternatively, other procedures such as IVs and bone marrow aspirations may be highly invasive, painful, and anxiety provoking and may be part of the diagnosis and treatment of life-threatening illnesses such as cancer. Procedures also include a range of interventions conducted in the course of acute (e.g., emergency department), routine (e.g., subspecialty outpatient), and intensive (e.g., intensive care or transplantation units) care.

The pain and distress associated with procedures in pediatric health care are one of the strongest areas of intervention science in pediatric psychology. Interventions for helping children, families, and staff prepare and cope with procedures have emerged from a strong tradition of behavioral research and have been successfully incorporated into treatment protocols, most often relying heavily on cognitive-behavioral approaches. Indeed, as Powers (1999) concludes from his review of 13 treatment outcome studies, CBT is a well-established treatment in pediatric psychology. The approaches used in protocols for procedural pain are quite diverse, including relaxation, breathing exercises, distraction, imagery, modeling, reinforcement, rehearsal, and coaching (Powers, 1999) and vary according to the age of the child.

There have been a few noteworthy shifts in pediatric practice related to procedures that affect the utilization of these highly effective psychological approaches. In the past decade, more effective pharmacologic support has been provided for children undergoing invasive procedures. In part related to increased attention to pain and the availability of safe and effective analgesics, conscious sedation and general anesthesia are both used more regularly, particularly for children with cancer and other procedure-intensive diseases (Zempsky, Schechter, Altman, & Weisman, 2004). Therefore, in most pediatric oncology treatment centers, pharmacologic approaches have become the front-line approach for helping children with procedural distress. Another change in practice relates to increasing use of surgically implanted central venous access catheters for children who would otherwise need repeated IV lines inserted, a practice associated with fewer reports of pain and anxiety (Slifer, Tucker, & Dahlquist, 2002). Another improvement in pediatric care that helps to reduce the pain and distress associated with needle sticks has been the accepted use of topical anesthetic creams that are longer acting than previous local anesthetics and are applied an hour or so in advance of the procedure.

Despite these shifts in practice, psychological interventions for procedural pain continue to have important roles in practice. For example, there is evidence that combined pharmacologic and psychologic interventions for procedural pain are effective and, in combination, may be more effective than either approach singly in preventing or reducing physiological pain pathways while enhancing self-efficacy and self-regulation of pain and distress (Kazak & Kunin-Batson, 2001; Kuppenheimer & Brown, 2002). In addition, for highly anxious children whose threshold for pain may be low, or for those who have learned maladaptive responses to procedures, psychological interventions offer important ways in which children and families can gain skills to cope with their distress. In other situations, pharmacologic interventions may not be feasible or acceptable to the child or family if needed regularly. There is also evidence that a psychosocial intervention may be helpful in reducing negative memories about procedures even in the absence of differences in immediate behavioral outcomes (Cohen et al., 2001). Finally, the cognitive-behavioral techniques that are effective for invasive procedures can be applied to less invasive procedures and to other diseases and circumstances where pain and anxiety are common reactions.

Intervention Studies for Pediatric Procedural Pain Published Since 1999

Recent outcome studies of cognitive-behavioral approaches to procedural pain continue to support the use of these approaches as effective treatments. In pediatric oncology, three newer papers by the same research group support the use of distraction for younger pediatric oncology patients and offer further support for the involvement of parents in a briefer protocol (Dahlquist, Busby, et al., 2002; Dahlquist, Pendley, Landthrip, Jones, & Steuber, 2002; Pringle et al., 2001). Chen, Craske, Katz, Schwartz, and Zeltzer (2000) also provide additional support for cognitive-behavioral intervention in children with leukemia and highlight the potential importance of targeting psychological interventions to those children with higher levels of pain sensitivity (Chen, Craske, et al., 2000).

The Dahlquist research group developed a 23-session distraction intervention, in which parents were taught the distraction procedure, that proved effective for five of eight young children with cancer (Pringle et al., 2001). In order to improve portability, this research group then tested a nine-session version of the protocol (Dahlquist, Busby, et al., 2002). Three different distractors were used in the study based on the age of the child: an electronic toy that prompts young children to find animals, shapes, and numbers; an 11-inch robot that speaks when the child correctly completes a matching task; and a toy laptop computer with 22 learning activities with a variety of sound effects and animals. The effects of this abbreviated treatment protocol were comparable to the 23-session protocol for five of six children. In the third study, Dahlquist, Pendley et al. (2002) used a Texas Instruments Touch & Discover electronic toy in the distraction intervention. This toy has several pictures depicting scenes attractive to preschoolers, such as barnyard animals and household objects. Mickey Mouse speaks, directing the child to press a picture, and each picture makes a sound. The picture panels vary in their degree of difficulty. Parents held the toy so that it blocked the child's view of the needle and prompted their child to play with the toy. Dahlquist and colleagues note that this distraction technique had effects to comparable those of other programs with much more involved parent training. Dahlquist and colleagues review the use of such a developmentally appropriate, multisensory distraction requiring both active cognitive processing and motor skills as an important factor in the success of their intervention.

Another study also examined the variable efficacy of different distractions. Mason, Johnson, and Woolley (1999) compared a cartoon to a short story as distractors for young children 2 to 4 years of age. Children would pick from a sample of cartoons, and parents encouraged the child to watch the cartoon during the procedure. In the storybook condition, parents read a storybook selected by the child and encouraged the child to press small pictures on the book that produced an associated sound. The short story procedure was more effective than the cartoon. Like the Touch & Discover toy used by Dahlquist and colleagues, this storybook required information processing, which may have reduced the capacity to process pain signals (Mason et al., 1999), as well as motor skill involvement. Mason et al. (1999) note that the storybook seemed to hold the attention of the child better than the cartoon and also may have helped calm parents by involving them more actively in helping their child cope with the needle. The calming of parents may have in turn helped calm the child. MacLaren and Cohen (in press), however, found that a cartoon distraction was more effective than an interactive toy condition in engaging the child and reducing distress during venipunctures for healthy children 1 to 7 years of age. MacLaren and Cohen suggest that children in the interactive toy condition might have become more bored with the distractor than those watching the cartoon. Alternatively, many children become anxious at the sight of the nurse, which may have interfered with their attention to the interactive toy compared to children watching the cartoon. Older children also seemed to be engaged more than younger children. Finally, MacLaren and Cohen suggest that their sample of healthy children may have been more distracted by the novelty of their environment compared to the Mason et al. (1999) sample of cancer patients who receive treatments routinely. The novelty may have interfered with their ability to focus on the toy distractor.

With respect to noncancer samples, Zelikovsky, Rodrigue, Gidycz, and Davis (2000) conducted a randomized clinical trial of a cognitive-behavioral intervention with 40 children, ages 3 to 7 years, undergoing a voiding cystourethrogram. Breathing exercises and tape-recorded positive statements were conceptualized as distraction and compared to standard care. For the breathing exercises, a party blower was used to teach these young children how to breathe deeply and slowly. Positive statements (e.g., "I can use my party blower to relax") were recorded and played during the medical procedure. These behavioral procedures were first modeled by the researcher and then practiced by the child and the child's parents, who were present during the actual medical procedure. Although pain and fear ratings were not associated with intervention condition, the intervention group evidenced less distress and more coping behaviors than did the control group.

In another study, a multicomponent cognitive-behavioral intervention was also shown to be effective in a single-group, repeated-measures design study of 43 children (mean age = 7 years) with human immunodeficiency virus (HIV) infection who were receiving venipunctures (Schiff, Holtz, Peterson, & Rakusan, 2001). The intervention was repeated for three injections, and a topical anesthetic was applied to the site of the injection, with its purpose explained to the child. The procedure itself was first performed on a doll. The researcher then modeled the coping procedure for the child and parent. Relaxation breathing was taught by blowing bubbles or blowing at a pinwheel. Other distraction devices were also offered, such as toys, books, and music, and the child was given a choice about distraction devices. Parents were instructed to coach the child's breathing and provide verbal reinforcement. The child practiced the procedure on a doll and then practiced as a patient. Children received stickers following the procedure. The first intervention training session took approximately 20 minutes, and the researcher coached the child through the procedure. The second session was a booster that reviewed the coping procedures. This session took about 10 minutes, and the parent was encouraged to be the primary coach during the actual procedure. In the third session, only reinforcement with stickers was provided. Observer ratings of behavioral distress, child-reported pain, and parent anxiety were found to decrease, although the lack of a comparison group affects interpretation of results.

Several recent papers highlight the potential value of distraction for reducing distress for preschooler and young children during immunization (Cassidy et al., 2002; Manimala, Blount, & Cohen, 2000) and IV insertion (Kleiber, Craft-Rosenberg, & Harper, 2001). All three studies used different approaches to distraction. Cassidy et al. (2002) compared the effectiveness of watching cartoons to watching a blank screen for injections and found that regardless of whether the TV was on or off, the distraction provided by looking at the TV resulted in less pain behavior. They concluded that a more potent or novel distraction than cartoon viewing is indicated. Kleiber et al. (2001) developed a 7-minute videotape in which three parents described why distraction was useful for their child. Key instructional points mentioned on the videotape included focusing the child away from the medical procedure, using activities (interactive books, blowing bubbles, novel toys, favorite stories), keeping the child focused on the parent, and praising the child at the end of the procedure. Both parents and children watched the video, and then children chose a distraction item to use during the procedure. Compared to standard care, parents in the experimental condition used significantly more distraction then did their counterparts. There was a trend for children in the experimental group to demonstrate reduced behavioral distress from IV insertion over time than did children in the standard care group.

Manimala et al. (2000) instructed parents to encourage their children to use a party blower prior to entering the treatment room and immediately prior to and during the procedure. The desired parent procedures and child coping behaviors were modeled to the parents and their children. The child pretended to receive the shot and was coached by the researcher and parent in the use of the party blower as a distractor. Results from a sample of 82 parent–child dyads assigned to either attention control, distraction, or reassurance conditions indicated that children in the distraction condition demonstrated the least amount of behavioral distress. Three times as many children in the reassurance condition than in the distraction condition required restraint by their parents during the injection.

Although each of the studies described above provides data that warrant careful consideration in the use of these techniques in this age group, the evidence for a consistent effect on pain or distress is mixed. In a study of 2- to 16-year-old patients ($N = 160$) undergoing IV insertion and randomized to distraction versus treatment as usual, distraction was not related to pain reduction but was seen as effective in reducing behavioral distress (Fanurik, Koh, & Schmidt, 2000). Distraction consisted of age-appropriate distraction techniques offered by the nurse and included bubbles and musical sound storybooks for the youngest age groups, sound storybooks and headsets with a choice of music for 9- to 12-year-olds, and listening to their choice of music using headphones for teenagers.

In summary, recent intervention studies in the area of procedural pain support the conclusions of Powers (1999) and lend further support to the use of cognitive-behavioral approaches as an empirically supported treatment for procedure-related pain. Distraction appears probably efficacious as an intervention for preschoolers, although its efficacy varies somewhat across types of distractors used (e.g., nonprocedural talk, cartoons, and interactive toys), across children within studies, and within children over time.

Using Distraction for Preschoolers in Clinical Practice

Distraction is currently the most commonly employed approach to helping preschoolers with procedure-related pain. Movies and cartoons have been the most commonly employed distractors in most studies. Sample guidelines for using distraction in practice, provided by Dr. Lindsey Cohen, are given in table 5.1 (see also Cohen 2004b). Many school-age children can benefit from coping skills self-management training. Brief protocols are typically used in practice. A sample self-management protocol by Dr. Cohen is provided in table 5.2 (see also Cohen 2004a).

The latest research by Dahlquist, Busby, et al. (2002) and Mason et al. (1999) suggest that a multisensory, age-appropriate toy is the most effective distractor. Dahlquist, Busby, et al. (2002) feel such distractors are better able to sustain children's interest over time than more passive distractors such as videotapes. The activity, however, must be matched to both the developmental and ability level of the child. Dahlquist, Busby, et al. (2002) note that, if the task is too difficult, children lose interest in the toy, and then its distraction value is negligible.

Disease-Related Pain

Treating pain associated with pediatric health conditions, both from the illness processes themselves and from pain associated with treatment, is a common and

Table 5.1. Guidelines for Using Distraction With Preschoolers

1. Repeatedly encourage the parents to get their child to attend to the distractor (movie, toy, etc.) the whole time that they are in the treatment room. Also, encourage the parents to play with the toys to distract their child.

2. Distract the child as much as possible the whole time that he or she is in the treatment room, including all of the time prior to and following the actual injections. Also, repeatedly engage the child in playing with toys or watching the video. Overdo and exaggerate distraction!

3. Distraction suggestions:
   a. Frequently point toward the movie or the toy
   b. Ask questions about the show, such as, "Who is the good guy?" "Did you see that?" "What's going to happen next?"
   c. Say "Watch the movie!" "Look over there!"

4. Overdo distractions and *refrain from engaging in nondistracting behaviors,* especially informing, comforting, reassuring, or apologizing.

Note. Adapted with permission from *Guidelines for Using Distraction With Preschoolers,* by L. Cohen (2004, unpublished protocol).

Table 5.2. Child Coping Skills Training for School-Age Children

Child coping skills training	Steps
Motivational rationale	*You are about to get a shot. The shot may hurt a bit, but we are going to teach you two special tricks that you can use when you feel scared or upset. Teenagers, adults, and famous sports stars like ice skaters and basketball players use these tricks when they feel scared or nervous. You can use these tricks anytime that you feel upset, like when you have a hard test in school or if you are being teased. If you do these tricks just right, you will have no problem with the shot today. Are you ready to learn the two special tricks?*
Deep breathing	*The first trick is called "deep breathing." Deep breathing relaxes the body and the mind. First, imagine that you are a super strong snake. Now, take a slow, deep breath. Now, let it out with a slow hissing sound. (pause) Good! Now do it again. (pause) Wow. You are really good at this! Do this before, during, and after the shot, and I will watch the videotape to see how it worked for you.*
Positive affirmation	*The second trick is called the "mantra." Can you say that? (pause) You will repeat a special sentence over and over. You should whisper it slowly. When you say it, you will feel good. You should say it at least 10 times in a row each time that you use it. The special sentence is "I'm calm and cool." Repeat it slowly 10 times for me. (pause) You look calm and cool! Good job! Do this and do the "snake breathing" before the shot, during the shot, and after the shot.*
Choosing a distraction	*You can use either deep breathing or your mantra, or switch back and forth, before, during, after the shot. What will you do? Which do you like better? Let me see you do both of them again so I can make sure that you know them and I know what to look for when I watch the videotape. Good! Make sure you do them the whole time that you go back for you shot. Can you do that? Good!*

Note. Adapted with permission from *Coping Skills Training for School Age Children*, by L. Cohen (2004, unpublished protocol).

important issue for pediatric psychologists. Disease-related pain is reported across a range of conditions, with the most frequently observed diseases being sickle cell disease (SCD), juvenile rheumatoid arthritis (JRA), and cancer. Walco et al. (1999) prepared a paper for the *JPP* Empirically Supported Treatments Series in which they concluded that there were few evidence-based approaches to this work. They concluded, however, that some approaches were promising, specifically, those relying on cognitive-behavioral approaches.

Intervention Studies of Disease-Related Pain Published Since 1999

Evidence for the use of a cognitive coping skills training approach to address pain in children with SCD is emerging. Karen Gil and her associates have developed an intervention protocol based on their prior work with adults with SCD (Gil et al., 1996, 2000). The two-session protocol involves teaching children deep breathing relaxation, imagery, and calming self-talk combined with homework (an audiotape, daily practice assignments, and a diary). The second session, 1 to 2 weeks subsequent to the first, reviews the material. Additional steps to the intervention include monthly telephone contacts to review use of coping strategies and problem solving related to their use (Gil et al., 2001).

In their initial randomized clinical trial of the intervention, 49 children with SCD from 1st through 12th grade were randomized to cognitive coping skills training or to a standard care condition. The treatment condition was associated with reductions in pain sensitivity, as assessed on a laboratory measure of pain intensity (Gil et al., 1997). A subsequent report from the same study analyzed data at a 1-month follow-up for 46 of the original sample. While not replicating the findings at posttest, the data indicated that children in the treatment group used more coping skills, although these did not necessary translate into more effective pain management (Gil et al., 2001). Importantly, however, treatment effects (use of coping strategies) were associated with fewer health care contacts and better school attendance and general functioning (Gil et al., 2001). Using the criteria from the *JPP* Empirically Supported Treatments Series papers, cognitive coping skills training can be considered a promising intervention. In another recent review of empirically supported psychosocial interventions for pain in SCD, this approach was classified as probably efficacious when Gil's work on both adults and children was considered (Chen, Cole, & Kato, 2004).

From Great Britain, Thomas, Wilson-Barnett, and Goodhart (1998) conducted a pilot study of 30 patients with SCD (ages 15–35 years) comparing weekly sessions of CBT with an attention control condition and with standard medical care, concluding that there were no significant differences across treatment conditions, although there were some very preliminary indications that the psychological treatment may affect the interrelated outcomes of pain, anxiety and depression, and health care utilization. These investigators subsequently conducted a randomized clinical trial of 82 patients 15 to 35 years of age comparing an eight-session intervention using CBT (including cognitive therapy, relaxation training, coping skills, and education) with an attention control condition and medical treatment alone

(Thomas, Gruen, & Shu, 2001). The data provide evidence for the short-term (6-month) reduction in health care costs for the CBT group, a finding not further supported at 12 months posttreatment (Thomas et al., 2001).

Powers, Mitchell, Graumlich, Byars, and Kalinyak (2002) conducted a pilot study of three children with SCD receiving intensive pain management skills training. The treatment consisted of six sessions of a group family-based cognitive-behavioral intervention, incorporating education and instruction in coping skills such as deep breathing, modeling, behavioral rehearsal, and development of individualized approaches for pain. These preliminary data further support the use of cognitive-behavioral approaches within a family context for the treatment of pain in SCD.

Juvenile primary fibromyalgia syndrome (JPFS) is an important area of pain, representing a type of pain that is difficult to treat, persistent, and associated with sleep and mood disorders. In terms of controlled studies with sufficient sample sizes to extract potential treatments, little prior evidence has been reported (Walco et al., 1999). Pilot data from a controlled study of 30 patients with JPFS compared coping skills training (CST) with self-monitoring, using a crossover design (Kashikar-Zuck, Swain, Jones, & Graham, in press). The CST intervention consisted of six sessions (weekly for the first month and biweekly for the second month), with parent participation in three of the sessions. Interventions included progressive muscle relaxation, distraction and activity pacing, cognitive therapy approaches for negative cognitions, and problem solving. Preliminary evidence for improvement in coping with pain, depressive symptoms, and functionality is reported.

Using CBT for Disease-Related Pain in Clinical Practice

Although CBT has not been shown to be a well-established treatment for disease-related pain, we review the general approach to managing disease-related pain that clinicians typically use. There is much overlap with the cognitive and behavioral strategies, particularly relaxation, used for other problems, specifically headaches and RAP. Consequently, we do not describe these procedures in detail but focus on five factors relatively specific to disease-related pain and refer to material covered in preceding sections.

First, one of the specific features of psychosocial interventions for disease-related pain is that they almost always are conducted within the context of a multidisciplinary team. A strong collaborative agreement between physician and psychologist in the treatment of pain secondary to a disease, such as SCD or JRA, is necessary. Education regarding the disease itself, the reasons for pain associated with the disease, and how medicine is used to treat disease, especially myths about the use of pain medications, is particularly important to cover thoroughly with children and their parents or caretakers. Although one might presume that families have a good knowledge of their child's disease, this may not always be the case, and review of this information can be very important in setting the stage for improved pain management. In some programs, the treating physician is incorporated into the protocol specifically to provide the educational component with a particular emphasis on explaining medications (e.g., Powers et al., 2002). Other physical methods for managing pain, such as heating pads and warm baths, are also often discussed, as well as ways to combine medications, physical methods, and psychological techniques to optimally manage pain (Powers et al., 2002).

Second, besides a greater emphasis on education, treatment protocols for disease-related pain also typically focus more attention on how to assess and record levels of pain. This emphasis relates to the common finding that many children poorly discriminate among different levels of pain. Because disease-related pain is typically only managed and not "cured," it is particularly important to assess levels of pain accurately so that children can begin to see slight improvements in their condition and increase their feelings of self-efficacy regarding pain management. In addition, because physicians typically provide guidelines on what medications and dosages to use for pain based on intensity (e.g., mild, moderate, or severe), accurate pain assessment plays a key role in deciding on the treatment to be delivered, when to contact the doctor about the child's pain, and what information to provide the doctor so that he or she can tailor recommendations for pain management. Children are instructed to tell adults when they are experiencing pain and to rate this pain as part of the assessment procedure. Parents, in turn, are taught how to manage pain at home given the child's report.

Third, relaxation training for disease-related pain is more challenging because the pain itself often interferes with the child's ability to concentrate on the relaxation procedure. Therefore, relaxation training is often more intensive, conducted over a number of weeks, and tailored more extensively according to the child's response and responsiveness. Imagery techniques often receive added emphasis in relaxation procedures for pain. Variants of hypnotic techniques, such as deepening, can be used to help strengthen the relaxation procedure. In a deepening image, the child is instructed to count, and with each number counted they become more deeply relaxed. Children can count using imagery techniques such as slowly counting waves lapping up against their toes at the beach, counting trees as they walk through woods, or counting houses as they ride their bicycle. Other images instruct the child to visualize a setting in which they have been pain-free or to visualize turning off a "pain switch" in one's body so that the pain diminishes (Walco, Varni, & Ilowite, 1992). Other techniques used in hypnosis that can apply in extended relaxation procedures are to use the term "discomfort" rather than "pain" (see chapter 3).

Clinicians often choose to only conduct relaxation training and practice during pain-free periods, or during periods of lower pain intensity, during the first month of treatment because premature, unsuccessful attempts to use relaxation during a pain episode may result in the child feeling discouraged and unwilling to continue relaxation training. In addition, relaxation training is also used to help children cope with anxiety that may arise as they anticipate the onset of a pain episode. Parents, too, may be taught an abbreviated relaxation procedure to help them manage their own anxiety as they see their child struggle with a pain episode (Powers et al., 2002).

Fourth, in addition to relaxation, distraction techniques are taught to children with disease-related pain. Because many children with disease-related pain have frequent pain episodes, it is not always feasible—or recommended—to ask the child to use relaxation on all occasions of a pain episode. Thus, distraction techniques are specifically incorporated into pain-coping protocols. Like relaxation, distraction is presented as an active coping technique. Distraction techniques vary according to the child's preferences but may include listening to music, playing computer games, and so forth. Distraction techniques should be practiced in sessions and used at home.

And fifth, positive self-talk in disease-related pain includes not only statements about the child's self-efficacy in managing pain but also a review of the various steps in the child's pain self-management plan. An emphasis is placed on changing self-statements such that pain is viewed as manageable, rather than overwhelming, and that the child can actively help manage the pain rather than viewing himself or herself as a passive recipient of pain. Equally important is for the child to attribute successful outcomes to his or her active efforts at coping rather than simply passive relief secondary to medications or a natural waning of his or her disease-related pain.

6 Adherence

Issues related to treatment adherence in pediatrics are very common—at least some missed medications or lapses in following medication, diet, or other lifestyle recommendations may be the rule and not the exception. Estimates of nonadherence specific to pediatric chronic illness vary widely, although reports in the range of 40% to 60% are common (e.g., Riekert & Drotar, 2000, p. 4). Notable as well are recent data documenting nonadherence in life-threatening illnesses, such as pediatric cancer (Kennard et al., 2004; O'Riordan et al., 2004).

The consequences of nonadherence are serious and far-reaching. For example, increased morbidity (disease symptoms and complications) or mortality may result. In addition, higher rates of health care utilization (e.g., more outpatient and inpatient hospital visits) may be associated with nonadherence. Outcomes of clinical trials may also be affected, potentially rendering inaccurate data on the types and doses of interventions necessary for disease treatment and outcomes. Adherence is also inherently complex and intertwined with illness and treatment as well as individual, family, health care staff, and societal factors.

In the *Journal of Pediatric Psychology*'s Empirically Supported Treatments Series, interventions related to adherence in three conditions—asthma, juvenile rheumatoid arthritis (JRA), and type 1 diabetes—were reviewed (Lemanek, Kamps, & Chung, 2001). Pediatric obesity, another condition in which adherence to treatment recommendations is essential, was addressed in a separate paper in the series (Jelalian & Saelens, 1999). Unfortunately, there were no adherence interventions that met criteria for a well-established treatment across asthma, JRA, or diabetes. There were, however, several probably efficacious adherence interventions, including organizational strategies (e.g., changing clinic routines, simplifying treatment regimens) for asthma, behavioral approaches for JRA, and multicomponent and behavioral approaches for diabetes. With respect to childhood obesity, there are well-established treatments based on behavioral and multicomponent approaches for children and preadolescents, but not for adolescents (Jelalian & Saelens, 1999). The success of these interventions for childhood obesity implies that these families adhered to the diet and exercise recommendations that comprise the intervention protocol.

Intervention Studies of Pediatric Adherence Published Since 2001

In providing an update on interventions related to adherence, we have not restricted our search to particular illnesses or treatment regimens. Interventions that relate to adherence to treatment for diet and exercise in cystic fibrosis (CF) are described in detail in chapter 10. Two manuals for interventions, one developed by Lori Stark to increase calorie consumption and the other by Alexandra Quittner related to chest physiotherapy and medication adherence, are available to readers at the companion Web site for this book. In general, very few empirical data exist to support the use of particular adherence-enhancing treatment approaches. Recent reports on intervention studies for JRA (one study) and asthma (three studies) are summarized. The concluding section of this chapter addresses some of the challenges evident in this important area of work.

A randomized clinical trial for children and adolescents with JRA was conducted by Rapoff et al. (2002). Patients and parents in the treatment group ($N = 19$) completed a 30-minute intervention conducted by a nurse. The intervention was based on behavioral analytic approaches, focusing on prompts and reinforcers for taking medication, and included a 10-minute video and a booklet describing ways to enhance adherence. Four strategies were described: pairing medication taking with a well-established behavior such as tooth brushing (cueing), using a calendar to track and a record medication taking (monitoring), praising and rewarding adherence to taking medication (positive reinforcement), and using a punishment procedure such as time-out for refusal to take medication (discipline). A nurse reviewed the content of the study materials with the families. The control group ($N = 15$) received a general educational intervention, including a video on medical aspects of JRA and standard educational booklets about JRA, medications, and side effects. Both groups received follow-up phone calls for 1 year. A Group × Time interaction showed support for patients in the intervention arm, using electronic monitoring devices to assess adherence with medication at 1 year. There was no difference between the groups for changes in disease activity or for functional ability.

Noteworthy in part for its testing of a model of change in adherence, Bonner et al. (2002) conducted a randomized clinical trial of an intervention tested with an urban Latino and African-American sample of children and adolescents with asthma. The conceptual model, based on a stages of change framework, posits that there are four phases of readiness for adherence to asthma treatments: symptom avoidance (i.e., family refusal to recognize asthma as chronic disease and responding only to acute exacerbations), asthma acceptance (i.e., acceptance of the disease but responding to symptoms, not taking preventive steps), compliance (i.e., using prevention strategies but seeing changes in asthma symptomatology as treatment failures), and self-regulation (i.e., use of an action plan to address changes in symptomatology with input from the physician). Each phase incorporates a family model of responsibility—for example, the family does not recognize asthma as a chronic disease, the family takes action when symptoms change, and so forth.

Families were randomized to the intervention ($N = 56$) or control (usual medical care, $N = 63$) arm. A bilingual college-educated family coordinator delivered the intensive intervention by taking the role of educator for the family about asthma and its management, and facilitator of the relationships among the patient, family, and staff. The coordinator provided support for the families in monitoring the child's asthma, helping them interpret diaries and coaching them to present their diaries to their doctors. The intervention also included three educational workshops for groups of families, at 1-month intervals. The workshops focused on teaching families about the use of peak flow meters, using asthma diaries and interpreting the diary data to gauge effectiveness of medication use, and pharmacotherapy management. The overarching goal of the workshops was to impress upon parents the chronicity of asthma. The family coordinator had additional contacts with families by phone and helped them formulate questions for their medical appointments. In addition, the family coordinator made two home visits to each family and accompanied families to one or two doctor visits. For a group of eight or nine families, the family coordinator spent 12 to 14 hours on the phone, with average calls lasting about 30 minutes. A number of differences between the groups, all favoring outcomes for the intervention group, are reported. These include knowledge of asthma, health beliefs, self-efficacy, attainment of Phase 3 (compliance) or Phase 4 (self-regulation) of readiness, and use of appropriate medication strategies.

Two recent presentations highlight data emerging for two adherence interventions related to pediatric asthma. In one, 15 children 7 to 12 years old with asthma and their parents were randomized to an "adherence improvement" intervention group that used education, monitoring, and review of adherence data or to an education-only arm (Kamps, Rapoff, & Roberts, 2004). The adherence intervention was delivered at home for 6 weeks with a 2-week follow-up. The small sample was analyzed as a series of case studies, with results showing improvements in electronically monitored adherence in the treatment group. Other outcomes, including pulmonary function, quality of life, and health care costs, showed improvements for both groups, with no differential impact for the behavioral intervention condition (Kamps et al., 2004).

The second project, based on 44 youths 9 to 15 years old with asthma, tested a parent–youth "teamwork collaboration" against asthma education and standard care (C. Adams, Dreyer, Dinakar, & Portnoy, 2004). The four-session teamwork intervention, similar to the work of Anderson, Brackett, Ho, and Laffel (2000; see chapter 4 for details) built on the importance of engaging parents in the process of improving adherence and addressing important developmental issues regarding adolescent autonomy and conflict with parents, particularly those related to treatment adherence. The results provide preliminary evidence for the inclusion of teamwork interventions for enhancing adherence to treatment. Improvements in other outcomes were less evident, although several factors showed improvement regardless of condition (e.g., health outcomes, parent–child conflict).

Using Family Therapy Techniques With Adolescents in Clinical Practice

Normal developmental processes suggest that nonadherence will be encountered at some point in adolescence. Parent–adolescent conflict can also play a role in both initiating and maintaining nonadherence. As adolescents with a chronic disease become more and more independent, they will seek to gain more control over managing their illness. Some parents may be willing to let their adolescent assume greater autonomy in disease management, but many are hesitant to give up control, fearing their adolescent's medical condition might worsen. This situation can lead to tension in the family, which in turn affects adherence. Given these issues, family-centered therapy techniques have been commonly used in both research studies (e.g., Satin, La Greca, Zigo, & Skyler, 1989) and clinical practice to address issues related to adolescent nonadherence. For example, Wysocki et al. (2000) use four major techniques in their behavioral family systems therapy for adolescents with diabetes: communication skills training, problem-solving training, cognitive restructuring, and functional and structural family therapy interventions. Although these family therapy approaches have not been established as effective for the problem of nonadherence, they are considered promising treatments. In addition, these approaches are frequently used for other adolescent problems. Consequently, family problem-solving and communication techniques, including the use of emotional regulation in family discussions, are described here. These techniques can be used to manage typical parent–child and parent–adolescent conflict or adapted to a disease management issue. Use of these techniques specifically for adherence to CF medical regimen is described in chapter 10 and on the Web site for this book.

As a prelude to working with families, it is often useful to provide parents with information on normal adolescent development and then relate developmental issues to the problem of adolescent nonadherence. Below is a script for covering these points adapted from Steinberg and Levine (1990).

Normalizing Adolescent Rebellion

State: *When children become teenagers, they typically want to be on their own, which often leads to increased parent–teenager conflict. This increase in tension is normal, as is your child questioning your rules. At the same time, peers become more important to teenagers and take your place as experts. Before this, your child probably looked to you for advice and you had the final say. Your teenager's desire to make his or her own decisions can result in arguments, secrecy, and silence.*

The handout "What to Expect From Your Teenager" (table 6.1) contains information on behaviors that can be expected from teenagers. These situations should be reviewed with the parents and the ones particularly relevant to the family discussed.

Provide General Information on How to Respond to Adolescents
State: *Most parents have mixed feelings about their child's independence. As teenagers become older, negotiation and compromise will be necessary and often difficult. Being a parent also fulfills our own needs, to be in control, to be correct, and to be needed. It is easy to feel rejected when your teenager becomes independent.*

Table 6.1.   What to Expect From Your Teenager

Teenagers often view being close to parents as "babyish."
  They will often reject your efforts to be helpful, reassuring, or affectionate.
  "Don't touch me" doesn't mean go away; it just means the rules are changing.

Teenagers don't want to be seen with their parents.
  They want to look older and more independent.
  It may help to have your child bring a friend, sit separately, choose a place that is
  not a school hangout, and allow your child to stay home periodically.

Teenagers have a need for emotional and physical privacy.
  Teenagers guard their personal lives.
  Keeping thoughts and feelings to themselves establishes emotional
  independence.
  This does not necessarily mean your child is hiding misbehavior.

Teenagers will look for and find their parents' weaknesses.
  De-idealizing parents is part of establishing independence.
  Making parents appear "less perfect" makes becoming an adult less scary.
  Teenagers will point out your faults and idealize other adults.

Teenagers will often choose friends over family.
  Parents often have to bargain for time with their teenager.
  This is part of learning about new attitudes, behavior, styles, etc.

Teenagers turn everyday decisions into tests of their competence and your trust.
  Teens and parents have different opinions about what the teen should do.
  Underlying disputes are questions regarding the teenager's right to make inde-
  pendent decisions.
  Disputes are often about whether you think your child is mature enough to
  decide how to schedule his or her own activities and accept consequences.

Note. Based on material in *You and Your Adolescent: A Parent's Guide for Ages 10 to 20*,
by L. Steinberg and A. Levine, pp. 151–152, 1990.

Parents want to keep their teenager from making the same mistakes that they made and think they can guide them down a path that is likely to lead to success. Parents often feel hurt and unappreciated when their teenagers do not accept their advice and make independent decisions, often contrary to those we recommend.

The handout "How to Respond to Your Teenager" (table 6.2) contains a list of ways that parents can help manage feelings related to their teenager's behaviors. It also provides guidelines on how parents can allow their teenagers to grow independent without losing parental control or permitting exposure to danger. Review the handout with the parents and discuss their reactions to the information. In families with two parents, encourage them to use one another as a source of support in applying these techniques. Also be sure to share that it is very important that they *both* follow these same procedures.

Table 6.2.   How to Respond to Your Teenager

Don't take your teenagers steps toward independence personally.
   Your child is reacting to your role as a parent.
   Your child will challenge you no matter how fair you have been.

Allow rebellion within limits.
   Teenagers learn to make choices by having choices.
   It is important to allow teens to solve their problems and make small mistakes.
   It is important for parents to protect their teenagers from making mistakes that
   will cause irreparable damage.

Allow freedom to make some decisions but be clear about standards.
   Choose areas that you will allow your teen to make his or her own decisions.
      Clothing, decorating room, music, when homework is done
   Be clear about standards your child is expected to meet when making decisions.
      Clothes not skimpy or dirty
      Music not played too loud
      If homework falls behind then part of the weekend is spent catching up
   Match your level of control to your teenager's level of maturity.

Expect some mistakes.
   All teenagers make foolish decisions.
   Teenagers may not recognize when they are being manipulated.
   Teenagers may not ask for advice because it will make them seem less independent.
   It's important not to get angry or criticize them for poor judgment ("How could you
   be so stupid") because it will further undermine their confidence in themselves.
   Teach them that "everyone makes mistakes" and the best you can do is learn
   from the experience so that the same mistake is not made in the future.
   When you think your teenager is going to make a poor decision, use questions
   instead of judgments. This will help steer your teen from making a bad choice
   and not push him or her to stick with the poor choice to assert independence.
      "Is there another way to solve this problem?"
      "How will you feel about this decision a week from now?"

Don't be afraid to say no.
   Setting limits shows that you care.
   Teens turn to their friends for advice when parents do not set rules.
   Good rule. Say "yes" when you can and "no" when you have to.
      Safety issues are nonnegotiable (e.g., parties without adult supervision, drinking
      at a friend's house, walking home late at night)
   Don't cut off discussion even if the answer is "no."
      Debating controversial issues such as drugs and sex with parents helps teens
      adopt their own values instead of assuming their peers.

Note. Based on material in *You and Your Adolescent: A Parent's Guide for Ages 10 to 20,* by L. Steinberg and A. Levine, pp. 154–156, 1990.

Concluding Remarks to Parents

State: *I would like to go over a few final tips that can be used when engaging in a discussion with your teenager. First, be sure to show disapproval of your child's behavior, not your child. Don't criticize his or her personality or character. For example, instead of saying, "You are a selfish person," you might say, "That was a selfish thing to do." Or, instead of saying, "You are a liar," you might say, "It was wrong to lie to me." Then apply logical consequences if appropriate.*

And second, there may be times when you do end up saying hurtful things to your teenager. All parents do at some point. If this does happen, it is very important to talk with your child afterward and apologize. As much as your teenager appears to disregard your opinion, he or she still listens to what you say and will take these statements to heart. This can lead to feelings of low self-esteem and contribute to depression and other problems. Also remember that your teenager will model your behaviors. As much as you can, try to show your child behaviors that you would like him or her to imitate.

Family Communication

Communication among family members is a prerequisite to most if not all work with families, such as problem-solving training. The importance of being able to discuss issues in a simple, effective, and open fashion must be stressed to the family. The family needs to understand how miscommunication will interfere with their ability to discuss and solve family problems. It is important to emphasize that even families with good communication skills can improve and that it is very common for families to have at least some problem in communicating effectively. Quittner, Drotar, Ievers-Landis, and Hoffman (2004), in the manual available on the companion Web site to this book, give extensive guidelines about family communication that the reader is encouraged to review. Below are some simple guidelines on how to implement family communication training. These guidelines are adapted from Robin and Foster (1984)[1]:

I. Introduce active listening skills
   A. Discuss how solving problems together can be difficult
      because everyone in the family may have different feelings
      and ideas about the problem.

---

1. This material is taken from "Problem-Solving Communication Training: A Behavioral–Family Systems Approach to Parent–Adolescent Conflict," by A. L. Robin and S. L. Foster, in P. A. Karoly and J. J. Steffen (Eds.), *Adolescent Behavior Disorders: Foundations and Contemporary Concerns*, pp. 211–212, 1984, Lexington, MA: D. C. Heath. Copyright 1984. Used with permission.

B. Discuss strategies for making a statement.
   1. Make your statement *clear* and *short*—don't lecture.
   2. Don't call someone names or put them down
      (e.g., "You're lazy!").
   3. *Take* responsibility for your part in the problem
      (e.g., "I'm upset that you forgot to take your enzymes,
      but I know that I said I'd put some in your bag and
      didn't").
   4. Mix *supportive* statements with criticism (e.g., "While
      I'm glad you told me the truth, I'm still upset that you
      didn't take your enzymes").
   5. Provide an alternative behavior when being critical of
      another family member (e.g., "I wish you'd ask me
      nicely to do my treatments rather than ordering me to
      do them").
C. Introduce "active listening" skills as a strategy to use
   during problem solving to help make it easier to express
   differences in opinion, and present the three rules of active
   listening.
   1. Pay attention and don't interrupt until the family
      member completes the statement.
   2. Be neutral about the other person's views (think of
      them as neither good nor bad). Try to stay calm if you
      disagree.
   3. Restate the sender's messages in your own words.
   4. Begin restatements with phrases such as "I hear you
      saying that . . . ," or "You said you feel . . ."
D. Role-play active listening skills. Have the adolescent describe
   a problem and demonstrate the use of active listening skills
   for the family. Then have the parents practice active listening
   skills with the adolescent through role-play.
E. Elicit reactions from the adolescent and his or her family,
   and discuss the importance of using active listening skills.
II. Review negative and positive communication behaviors.
   A. Distribute and review the "Communication Guidelines"
      handout (table 6.3).

Table 6.3. Communication Guidelines

Problematic behavior	Possible alternatives
Accusing/blaming	Make "I" statements (I feel ____ when ____ happens)
Put-downs/criticizing	Make "I" statements, note good and bad
Interrupting	Listen, take turns
Overgeneralizing/ catastrophizing	Make accurate statements
Lecturing/preaching	Make brief, problem-oriented statements
Sarcastic tone	Use a neutral tone of voice
Looking away	Make eye contact
Mind reading	Ask questions, don't assume
Give commands	Give rationale and then ask nicely (please)
Dwelling on past	Stick to present and future
Monopolizing the conversation	Take turns
Threatening	Give *realistic* alternatives that can be carried out
Remaining silent	Share your feelings
Yelling/swearing	Separate, cool down, re-engage when ready using respectful language and a normal tone of voice

Note. Adapted from "Problem-Solving Communication Training: A Behavioral–Family Systems Approach to Parent–Adolescent Conflict," by A. L. Robin and S. L. Foster, in P. A. Karoly and J. J. Steffen (Eds.), *Adolescent Behavior Disorders: Foundations and Contemporary Concerns,* pp. 211–212, 1984, Lexington, MA: D. C. Heath. Copyright 1984. Used with permission.

    B. Review negative communication habits and engage in a discussion about those used by the adolescent and his or her parents or guardians.

    C. Review positive communication habits and engage in a discussion about how they can replace negative communication styles.

    D. Discuss the negative or hurtful effects of negative communication behaviors (e.g., can invoke anger, resentment, low self-esteem, etc.).

  III. Discuss the importance of emotion regulation and review related strategies. Inevitably, there will be times when parents lose their temper with their adolescent. Therefore, it is important to review with parents' ways to maintain control when dealing with their adolescent. The same can be said for adolescents when dealing with their parents. Described here are some techniques for helping parents or guardians to remain calm.

   A. Briefly review potential strategies that can be used by the adolescent and their parents or guardians to calm down prior to engaging in discussions. Distribute and review the "Parent Emotion Regulation Techniques" handout (table 6.4).

   B. Review the importance of not forcing anyone to engage in a discussion when the parties are not ready or upset. If a discussion that initially starts off in a calm tone becomes heated, separate and give one another adequate time to cool off. *Do not* re-engage in the discussion until both parties are ready.

Family Problem Solving

There are a number of different problem-solving systems that can be found in the literature. Below is an example of a problem-solving approach entitled

---

Table 6.4.   Parent Emotion Regulation Techniques

1. State that you need to take a "time out" and leave the scene.

2. Take steps to help yourself calm down, such as counting to 10, telling yourself to relax, and taking a few deep breaths.

3. After you have calmed down, think about the situation:
   All teenagers make mistakes and disobey their parents.
   I don't have to scream for my child to know how upset I am.
   I am not an awful, inadequate parent if my child misbehaves.
   This does not mean that my child doesn't respect or care about me.
   This does not mean my child will grow up to be a delinquent.
   It's disappointing when my child misbehaves, but I can handle it.
   I can show my disapproval calmly and still get rid of my anger.
   Am I expecting too much of my child?

4. After assessing the situation calmly, think about your options:
   What can I do to handle this situation calmly and fairly?
   Which options seems best?

5. After you try to resolve the problem:
   You may not be able to completely resolve the conflict at that time and may still feel angry. Remember, no child or parent is perfect, but you are working on making things better. Thinking about it over and over again only makes you more upset. If you succeed in solving the problem, congratulate yourself. You might tell yourself, "I handled that pretty well. I could have gotten more upset than it was worth, but I actually got through it without losing my cool."

Note. Based on material in *Instructor's Manual for the Adolescent Coping With Depression Course,* by G. Clarke, P. Lewinsohn, and H. Hops, 1990; and *Treating Alcohol Dependence: A Coping Skills Training Guide* (2nd ed.), by P. M. Monti, R. Kadden, D. J. Rohsenow, N. Cooney, and D. Abrams, 2002.

"SOLVE" (Donaldson, Spirito, & Overholser, 2003), which is also described in chapter 3 for use individually with adolescents:

The SOLVE system (Donaldson et al., 2003) consists of the five problem-solving steps that correspond to each letter in the acronym. These steps are described below. Table 6.5 presents a worksheet that can be used when completing the SOLVE system.

"S" = Select a Problem
Discuss rules for defining the problem (Clarke, Lewinsohn, & Hops, 1990):

Table 6.5.   Family Problem-Solving Worksheet

Name:
Date:
Select problem:

Options	Likely Outcome (+, −, +/−)		
	Teen	Mom	Dad
1. _____			
2. _____			
3. _____			
4. _____			
5. _____			
6. _____			
7. _____			
8. _____			

Circle the Very Best One

Evaluate: How well did it work?

1	2	3	4	5
not well			very well	

Note. Adapted from *Instructor's Manual for the Adolescent Coping With Depression Course,* by G. Clarke, P. Lewinsohn, and H. Hops, p. 12.4, 1990, Portland, OR: Kaiser Permanente Center for Health Research, http://www.kpchr.org/public/acwd/acwde.html. Used with permission.

1. Begin with something positive.
2. Be specific.
3. Describe what the other person is doing or saying that is problematic.
4. Do not engage in name-calling when describing the problem.
5. Express your feelings in reaction to the problem.
6. Admit your contribution to the problem.
7. Don't blame others.
8. Be brief.

"O" = Options

After everyone agrees on the problem and understands it, all possible solutions to the problem should be generated. Family members should be assisted in withholding judgments of the different options.

"L" = Likely Outcomes

Each person rates the outcomes with a plus or minus.

"V" = Very Best One to Do

Family members identify the solution that seems most acceptable to everyone.

"E" = Evaluate and Repeat Process as Necessary

The therapist assists the family in reviewing the SOLVE problem-solving system. If the adolescent has previously learned parts or all of the steps, the adolescent may be asked to assist the therapist in teaching the problem-solving steps to their parents or guardians. The problem-solving process is commonly affected by family members interrupting each other, not paying attention to other family members, and criticizing an idea generated by another family member. Therapists typically develop rules around these behaviors at the beginning of a family problem-solving session to circumvent these problems in the exercise. Communication training also helps address these potential problems.

The therapist and family members conclude the session by discussing the importance of evaluating the outcome of the solution chosen and repeating the problem-solving process if the problem still exists. In the course of concluding a family problem-solving exercise, parent and adolescent beliefs and expectations about the exercise should be discussed. The therapist will often need to clarify expectations of both the parent and adolescent before progress can be made in the use of problem solving. The reader is referred to the manual, available on the companion Web site to this book, developed by Quittner, Drotar, Ievers-Landis, and Hoffman (2004), which contains a module on addressing beliefs held by parents and adolescents that can affect adherence to medical regimens, specifically CF. The Quittner et al. manual also gives more details, including dialogue on how to conduct a family problem-solving session.

Challenges to Adherence Interventions

Given the importance of adherence and the opportunities it affords for collaborative practice with physicians and nurses, the overall lack of effective treatments in this area is of significant concern. In order to promote dialogue and collaborative studies, we outline four general areas that represent challenges in the field.

The Limitations of Existing Language

The classic definition from which adherence work was derived was from R. Haynes (1979), discussing compliance as "the extent to which a person's behavior . . . coincides with medical or health advice" (pp. 2–3). The term *compliance* suggests a unilateral relationship (i.e., health care provider determines what patient should do) and assumes that the medical advice prescribed represents a "gold standard," which is understandable and important to the patient and family, reasonable to implement, and effective for all patients. While the term compliance continues to be used regularly in medical settings, the alternative term—*adherence*—is preferred by many health care researchers and providers. As Riekert and Drotar (2000, p. 7) note, adherence de-emphasizes patient and family obedience and highlights the critical active roles that patients and families play in treatment decisions. These issues are particularly salient in pediatrics where the child patient is generally inseparable from the family.

Others have used more specifically patient-oriented terms, such as self-care and disease management (La Greca, 1990) and self-regulation, self-change, and collaborative management (Creer, 2000). These models are more explicit about the importance of patient, family, health care team, school, and community in the collaborative pursuit of adaptive health outcomes (Power, DuPaul, Shapiro, & Kazak, 2003). The natural tensions between and among collaborative partners must be considered and addressed (e.g., parent–adolescent disagreements, frustrations experienced between physicians and families, pressures on health care providers to see more patients in less time, different agendas, and potential miscommunications between schools and families). All of these areas are ripe for intervention, although complex and difficult to tackle in intervention research.

Measurement Issues

Adherence is challenging to measure. Adherence is often conceptualized as whether a child has taken a medication or not. This is a simple dichotomous outcome that can overlook the complexity of care. For example, medication may need to be taken several times a day. Skipping a dose may be more or less significant, depending on the illness and its stage, and the patient may or may not understand this. A regimen might include multiple, interactive medications, possibly on an alternate dosing schedule. There may be conflicting (or unclear) directives for what the patient and family should do if a dose is missed, if the dosage is incorrect (too high, too low), or if the child is otherwise ill or unable to take a dose. Although thoughtful, multifaceted, and sophisticated measurement approaches to adherence continue to be developed, the outcomes from intervention studies will be limited if the measurement approaches are unreliable or invalid, from either a conceptual or a measurement perspective.

Beliefs and Culture

Most interventions to promote adherence understandably rely on the strong behavioral traditions of psychological interventions. Thus, similar to other areas of effective intervention, cognitive-behavioral and behavioral approaches are predominant and useful in inducing changes in behavior. In many situations, a sense of urgency—nonadherence could contribute to adverse medical outcomes—adds to the pressure for interventions that can be implemented in a nimble and individualized manner. Relatively little attention has been paid to the acceptability of adherence interventions to patients and families. One significant part of this is consideration of how family beliefs and cultural factors may influence the usefulness of adherence interventions.

For example, rather than focus on why some patients and families are not adherent, some authors raise the possibility that some noncompliance or experimentation is natural and not necessarily problematic. They ask questions such as, "Why be compliant?" "Why does anyone do what they are asked to do by their health care providers?" and "What are the patients' natural beliefs about treatment and their adherence?" (C. Adams, Joseph, et al., 2004; Deaton, 1985; Stein & Pontious, 1985).

It is also not uncommon to find, for example, that children and adolescents (and their families) may question certain aspects of treatment. It may be difficult, for example, for a child to see that chemotherapy that makes him or her ill in the short run will be helpful in the long term. Parents may feel that some treatments are more important than others and advocate less stringently for some components of the treatment protocol. Cultural, spiritual, and religious beliefs may be in direct conflict with medical recommendations (e.g., blood transfusions recommended in the case of Jehovah's Witnesses, or belief in complementary medicine approaches rather than standard treatment recommendations). In one of the few studies to examine adherence specifically in an ethnic minority group of pediatric patients, Tucker et al. (2001) reported differences in predictors of medication adherence in African-American renal transplantation patients compared with Caucasian patients. The data have interesting implications for adherence interventions. Interventions that provide cues and reminders may be more predictive of adherent outcomes for Caucasian patients than for African-American youths. The latter group's adherence was more strongly influenced by their motivation and self-efficacy than by prompts.

Broader Perspectives on Adherence

Most literature on adherence has focused on specific diseases and treatments, a logic that follows a medical model and the resulting organization of health care organizations. However, this compartmentalized approach may detract from opportunities to look at factors that influence adherence across conditions, families, and health care teams. Recent models have been proposed that can consider adherence as "multidimensional and dynamic, and involving a triadic partnership" (DeCivita & Dobkin, 2004, p. 158). There is strong support for the importance of families in adherence and for developing approaches that facilitate the collaborative joining of patient, family, and health care systems in formulating intervention approaches.

The importance of the family is evident in research on adherence in diabetes (Wysocki et al., 1999) and CF (DeLambo, Ievers-Landis, Drotar, & Quittner, 2004) and successfully incorporated in adherence interventions in these diseases. For example, behavioral family systems therapy explicitly focuses on parent–adolescent conflict related to disease management (Wysocki et al., 2000). Other interventions commonly utilize group intervention formats, often parents and children or teens separately, to focus on aspects of adherence specific to their roles. Looking across disease groups and thinking more broadly about families may lead to alternative ways to address adherence.

The work of Barbara Fiese and her colleagues looks at the role of family rituals in adherence to asthma. While it is widely accepted that pediatric illness and treatment regimens disrupt individual and family functioning, little attention has been paid explicitly to how these disruptions (and subsequent reorganizations) could be used to enhance our understanding of how families adhere to treatments. As proposed by Fiese and Wamboldt (2000), a decision tree can guide assessment related to routines, rituals, and adherence. When adherence is an issue, the family's routines should be explored. For the majority of families who have routines (i.e., rhythm and flow to how things get done at home and who does what), routines may become disrupted by the diagnosis of asthma. Families may benefit from redefining their routines and integrating treatment-related demands into them. For example, some of the most effective ways of prompting adherence to treatments that involve dietary recommendations are for the entire family to adopt at least some significant part of the diet. Those families without routines are generally seen as more problematic and more likely to have other difficulties in family functioning in addition to adherence. In these cases, Fiese and Wamboldt (2000) suggest identifying whether there is conflict around the need for a routine or whether routines need to be developed.

The eight-item Asthma Routines Questionnaire was developed and administered to 153 families with a child with asthma, yielding two factors, Medication Routines and Routine Burden (Fiese, Wamboldt, & Anbar, 2005). Medication Routines were associated with adherence and health care utilization, whereas Routine Burden was related to quality of life. The data are supportive of a brief screening approach that may direct the treatment team in the direction of asking about family routines associated with asthma adherence and helping to disentangle quality of life issues from adherence per se (Fiese et al., 2005).

In addition to conflict and family rituals, there is also evidence that parenting style affects adherence. Authoritative parenting (e.g., warmth, support, control) was associated with better adherence in preschool and school-age children with diabetes (Davis et al., 2001) than was other types of parenting. These data are quite intriguing when considered in combination with the evidence for parent–child conflict in diabetes management that has been described in adolescence (Jacobson et al., 1994).

School and peer influences on adherence represent another important area of work. There is a literature on school-based interventions of a primarily psychoeducational nature, but relatively less has been written on peer influences on adherence and the potential role of the school in facilitating adherence plans. Given the increasing complexity of children with pediatric illnesses who are attending school on a regular basis and the amount of time spent at school, facilitating linkages between the family, hospital, and school in terms of adherence is important. In the area of obesity, Jelalian and Mehlenbeck (2002) added peer-based skills training to a cognitive-behavioral group treatment intervention. Pilot data are supportive of the potential benefit of enhancing peer skills, with its potential contribution to weight loss and increase in self-confidence.

Power and colleagues propose a nine-step model, applicable for intervention approaches across systems (Power et al., 2003). These include the following:

1. *Identify the team.* Identify the key players from the family, hospital, and school, and establish specifically how they will work together.
2. *Establish goals.* Establish the goals for the intervention to increase adherence.
3. *Determine leadership.* In order to address complicated issues related to adherence across systems, clarify the leadership of the team.
4. *Communicate broadly.* Conveying information in a timely and succinct manner in terms of progress of the adherence plan is essential for success.
5. *Intervene strategically.* Use the best practices for the issue identified, and target the adherence intervention accordingly.
6. *Adjust plans.* A complex plan for adherence will need monitoring and adjustment.
7. *Resolve conflicts.* Conflicting information and opinions are natural in complex systems. Approaching conflict to resolve it is an adaptive orientation.
8. *Look ahead.* Once the immediate adherence concern is resolved, determine what lies ahead. An increasing number of children with serious illness are entering young adulthood, when unresolved issues related to adherence may continue to be problematic.
9. *Evaluate outcomes.* The need for outcomes on adherence intervention must ultimately include data about the usefulness of interventions implemented outside the research context. Evaluating the feasibility and achievement of goals is essential.

IV INTERVENTIONS FOR SPECIFIC DISORDERS

7 Nocturnal Enuresis

Nighttime bedwetting is experienced as part of normal development by virtually all young children. It is not until a child is 5 years of age, and the bedwetting occurs at least twice per week for at least 3 consecutive months, that a diagnosis of nocturnal enuresis is conferred (American Psychiatric Association, 1994). Approximately 10% of school-age children wet their beds, usually nightly (Jarvelin, Vikevainen-Tervonen, Moilanen, & Huttunen, 1988), and therefore qualify for the diagnosis. Although the rate of nocturnal enuresis declines with age, it usually takes several years before bedwetting spontaneously remits. Consequently, there has been a great deal of research examining whether behavioral treatment approaches can lead to more rapid elimination of bedwetting.

Mellon and McGrath (2000) reviewed the literature on behavioral treatment of nocturnal enuresis as part of the *Journal of Pediatric Psychology*'s Empirically Supported Treatments Series and found 39 studies to review. The treatment approaches used to address nocturnal enuresis in these studies were categorized as follows: urine alarms, urine alarms plus other behavioral treatments including multicomponent treatment such as Full-Spectrum Home Training (Houts & Liebert, 1984) and Dry Bed Training (Azrin, Sneed, & Foxx, 1974), combined medical/behavioral approaches, and psychological therapies including hypnosis.

In this chapter, we briefly review the findings of the Mellon and McGrath (2000) article and present summaries of recently published papers on the treatment of enuresis. The majority of this chapter focuses on urine alarms and urine alarms plus other behavioral treatments because they have received the most empirical support in the literature. Nonetheless, there are studies suggesting that medication [desmopressin (DDAVP)] plus urine alarms may be superior to urine alarms alone (Bradbury & Meadow, 1995; Sukhai, Mol, & Harris, 1989). This combined pharmacologic/behavioral approach may be particularly useful in addressing the bedwetting of children who have multiple episodes of bedwetting per night (Mellon & Houts, 1998).

Urine Alarms

A urine alarm refers to either a pad placed on the bed or a small moisture-sensing device attached to the child's underwear or pajamas. At the first detection of moisture, the battery-powered alarm rings near the child's ear. Mellon and McGrath (2000) cite a number of studies demonstrating that urine alarms are superior to psychotherapy and medication alone in treating enuresis. The findings are very consistent with an average success rate of about 78% for children treated with urine alarm systems (Mellon & McGrath, 2000); thus, urine alarms have been designated an effective treatment.

Studies Published on Urine Alarms Since 1999

A review of the literature since 1999 did not indicate any further studies examining the efficacy of urine alarms for the treatment of nocturnal enuresis. Indeed, the literature on urine alarms is so strong that there is probably no need to investigate efficacy unless there are substantial technical advances in the equipment that would then require validation.

Using Urine Alarm Protocols in Practice

There are a number of companies that manufacture urine alarms, but they all use essentially the same methodology. Clinicians should experiment with different alarms to find the one they like the best. The instructions by clinicians to parents/caregivers and from parents/caregivers to children regarding the use of the alarm are also important. The following guidelines, adapted from Schmitt (1987), may be useful.

1. Have the child hook up the alarm by himself or herself with parental supervision. The child should set off the alarm by touching the sensor with a wet finger and then practice going to the bathroom.
2. Use a night light or keep the bathroom light on overnight.
3. As soon as the alarm sounds, the child should stand up, deactivate the alarm, and go quickly to the bathroom. After urinating in the toilet, the child should put on dry underwear or pajamas, reconnect the alarm, with help from parents/caregivers if necessary, and put a towel over the wet spot on the bed.

4. Record wet and dry nights each morning.

5. When a child does not awaken at the sound of the alarm, parents/caregivers should go to the child's bedroom, turn on the lights, and loudly tell the child to get out of bed and stand up. If this approach fails, sit the child up in bed and place a cold washcloth on the child's face. When the child is standing up, remind the child to turn off the alarm. Make sure the child is awake and walks into the bathroom on his or her own. Asking the child questions is one approach that may help awaken the child. Follow these procedures until the child is able to wake on his or her own.

Urine Alarms in Combination With Behavioral Techniques

A number of researchers have examined whether the addition of behavioral techniques to urine alarms improves treatment efficacy (e.g., Bollard & Nettlebeck, 1981). Two of the best-known treatment packages are Full-Spectrum Home Training (Houts & Liebert, 1984) and Dry Bed Training (Azrin et al., 1974). Dry Bed Training meets the criteria for an effective treatment, whereas Full-Spectrum Home Training was classified as probably efficacious because it has not been replicated by a second investigator.

Full-Spectrum Home Training

Full-Spectrum Home Training uses a number of behavioral techniques to improve upon urine alarm training alone, including self-monitoring of wet and dry nights, retention control training with reinforcement, and overlearning. Self-monitoring is accomplished with a relatively simple chart that the child is asked to complete each morning with supervision from parents as necessary. Retention control training refers to a technique in which the child practices, during the daytime, restraining the urge to urinate for gradually longer periods until this control can be accomplished successfully for 45 minutes. The rationale that is communicated to parents/caregivers and the child is that the ability to hold more urine in the daytime may result in a similar increase in capacity at night. Parents/caregivers are instructed to give their child plenty to drink at a specific time of day. When the child wishes to urinate, parents/caregivers are instructed to encourage the child to wait a few minutes longer before going to the bathroom. Children are asked to urinate in a measuring cup so they can keep daily records of urine volume. Children are encouraged to complete the daily monitoring sheet by themselves and receive small rewards every day the previous volume record is improved upon.

The last component of Full-Spectrum Home Training, overlearning, begins after the child has attained 2 complete weeks of dry nights. At that point, the child is asked to drink larger and larger amounts of water before going to bed. The urine alarm continues in use until the child can attain 2 more complete dry weeks under these conditions. Mellon and McGrath (2000) cite three studies indicating that Full-Spectrum Home Training results in cure rates of 60% to 70%. However, these rates were not significantly superior to rates obtained using other approaches that also include urine alarms.

Dry Bed Training

Dry Bed Training has been described in detail in a self-help book by Azrin and Besalel (1979) entitled *A Parent's Guide to Bedwetting Control.* Dry Bed Training entails a waking schedule, the practice of appropriate toileting (Positive Practice), cleanliness training, and use of a urine alarm. On the first night, an intensive training period is conducted. One hour before bedtime, the urine alarm is placed on the bed, and then Positive Practice ensues. The child lies down on the bed, counts to 50, gets up, walks to the bathroom, and attempts to urinate. The child repeats this procedure 20 times. Just before bedtime, the child is asked to drink fluids. Hourly awakenings then occur throughout the night. After awakening, the child is asked to walk to the bathroom, guided by the parent if necessary. At the bathroom door, the child is asked to inhibit urinating if possible and is praised for doing so when this occurs. The child then returns to the bed, where he or she is asked to feel the sheets and state that they are dry. The child is praised for keeping the bed dry, given fluids to drink, asked to repeat instructions for the next hourly waking, and then returns to sleep. If the child is unable to inhibit urination but does perform the toileting routing appropriately, the child is praised for correct toileting. This occurs through-out the night. If a bedwetting accident occurs, the parent or caregiver disconnects the alarm, awakens the child, and takes the child to the bathroom to finish urinating. Cleanliness Training is then conducted. Cleanliness Training entails having the child change pajamas, remove the bedsheet and place it in the laundry, get clean sheets, and place the sheets on the bed. The alarm is then reconnected. Positive Practice is then performed, again 20 times, during the night.

After the first night of intensive training, a comparable but less intensive procedure is followed. If there has been an accident the prior night, the Positive Practice routine is enacted. The child is reminded to stay dry overnight and that Cleanliness Training and Positive Practice will occur overnight if wetting occurs. Before the parents/caregivers retire for the night, they wake the child and the child goes to the bathroom. After each dry night, the parents/caregivers awaken the child one half hour earlier than the night before. This awakening continues until the time falls within 1 hour of the child's bedtime. When accidents occur, Positive Practice and Cleanliness Training are implemented that night and the next evening before bed. After dry nights, the parents/caregivers praise the child frequently throughout the next day. After 7 consecutive dry nights, this procedure is discontinued. If one bedwetting incident occurs, the child receives Cleanliness Training that morning and Positive Practice at night prior to bed. If two accidents occur within 1 week, the entire training protocol is reinstated until 7 consecutive dry nights occur again.

Eight studies were reviewed by Mellon and McGrath (2000) and indicated that approximately three-quarters of children treated with this technique achieved complete cessation of wetting with a treatment protocol lasting 1 month on average. These studies demonstrated superiority of the dry bed method to treatments such as urine alarm alone and retention control training. Despite its success as a treatment, it has been noted that using Dry Bed Training without the urine alarm reduces its effectiveness (e.g., Keating, Butz, Burke, & Heimberg, 1983). In addition, Mellon and Houts (1998) raise concerns about the demanding nature of the program upon the child and family. Consequently, some would advocate that the urine alarm is sufficient treatment.

Studies on Urine Alarms in Combination With
Behavioral Techniques Published Since 1999

There have been no additional studies since the publication of the Mellon and McGrath (2000) article on the use of urine alarms plus behavioral techniques for enuresis. Thus, Dry Bed Training remains an effective treatment and Full Spectrum Home Training remains a probably efficacious treatment.

Psychological Treatments: Hypnosis

Hypnosis is the psychological treatment approach that has been used most commonly with enuresis. Mellon and McGrath (2000) cite four studies with an average success rate of approximately 70% achieved in an average of six sessions. However, only one of these studies was controlled, and that study did not quantify its outcome measures. The approach used in each of these studies was similar. First, there is an induction phase, followed by deep relaxation and then suggestion for achieving bedtime continence, either therapist directed or through self-hypnosis. Because the data supporting hypnosis do not clearly demonstrate efficacy and because hypnosis requires specialized training and practice in techniques beyond that typically obtained in professional training programs, hypnosis protocols are not described here.

New Approaches

Two variants of the urine alarm treatment protocol have been described. El-Anany, Maghraby, Shaker, and Abdel-Moneim (1999) randomly assigned 125 children with enuresis to one of two groups. In the first condition, parents/caregivers were instructed to have their children get up and void at a time when their bladder was full and they were still dry. In the second group, parents/caregivers were instructed to wake their children up after 2 or 3 hours of sleep, regardless of whether they were dry or wet. In the first group, parents determined the time to awaken the child based on a systematic method of waking the child up 3 hours after bedtime and either increasing or decreasing the time by 15 minutes depending on whether the child was wet or dry. This tailored "alarm clock" method was 77% successful at the end of treatment compared to 62% in the group with the set alarm time. The relapse rate was slightly better in the second group after 3 months (9% vs. 15%) and 6 months (15% vs. 24%). El-Anany et al. (1999) note that the tailored alarm procedure has the advantage over urine alarms in that the child does not have to wet in order for the treatment to be conducted.

Pretlow (1999) had children with enuresis wear a miniature bladder volume measurement instrument during sleep. The instrument automatically measured bladder volume every 15 minutes, and an alarm signaled when the bladder reached a specified volume. Children were assigned to two groups. In the first group, an alarm sounded when bladder volume reached 80% of the child's typical daytime voided volume, and in the second group, the alarm sounded at 80% of the typical nighttime enuretic volume. The treatment protocol lasted from 3 to 12 months for those who completed the protocol. In both groups, the mean dry night rates increased from less than one-third of nights dry to more than 80% dry nights. In both groups, nighttime bladder capacity increased about 70%. The cure rate was 55% in the first group after an average treatment length of 10.5 months and 60% in the latter group after an average of 7.2 months of treatment. Like the El-Anany et al. (1999) study, this approach has an advantage over urine alarms in that the conditioning occurs to a full bladder rather than to wetting. Nonetheless, both these approaches will need further testing before they become common in clinical practice.

Daytime biofeedback training has been suggested as an appropriate treatment for refractory nocturnal enuresis, especially when there are physiologic abnormalities. Hoekx, Wyndaele, and Vermandel (1998) treated 24 patients with nocturnal enuresis, small bladder capacity, and detrusor instability. Biofeedback was conducted weekly for 1 month and then daily for 2 weeks. A catheter was inserted into the bladder, and the bladder filled slowly until a detrusor contraction occurred. Patients were then asked to inhibit the contraction. Bedwetting was eliminated in 17 of 24 children after an average of about 8 weeks of treatment. Bladder capacity increased in all patients during treatment. Fifteen patients remained dry at night at 11-month follow-up.

Clinical Issues

The literature indicates that a urine alarm must be very strongly considered in any behavioral treatment of nocturnal enuresis. The recent study by El-Anany et al. (1999) suggests that the "alarm clock" procedure might prove a useful substitute for a urine alarm, but the two approaches have yet to be directly compared. Similarly, Pretlow's (1999) bladder volume measurement instrument might also be used in place of a urine alarm if comparative studies demonstrate its superiority over a urine alarm. The multicomponent approaches, such as Full-Spectrum Home Training, achieve slightly higher remission rates over urine alarms alone. Behavioral techniques also appear indicated as an addition to urine alarm protocols to help address relapse. The more intensive multicomponent approaches, such as Dry Bed Training, do not appear necessary to achieve results significantly better than less demanding multicomponent protocols. Medication is another possible treatment approach to prevent relapse and may prove necessary for certain conditions, such as multiple nighttime wetting.

When urine alarms are used, the manner in which clinicians describe the use of urine alarms is likely to affect acceptance by parents/caregivers and adherence to the procedure. Adequately preparing parents/caregivers for the intensive nature of the urine alarm program is also important. Although one parent/caregiver typically takes primary responsibility for the training, it is important to enlist other caregivers in the treatment, such another parent/partner, grandparents, or other adult family members living in the home. It is equally important to ensure that other family members do not interfere with program implementation. Kainz (2002) recommends that parents be instructed as follows:

- Stop all other behavioral treatments they may have tried in the past or are currently using (e.g., waking up the child in the middle of the night).
- Do not scold or punish the child for wetting the bed.
- Have the child maintain a regular bedtime and get sufficient sleep because fatigue makes training more difficult.

There are also a number of other helpful approaches to implementing the urine alarm procedure. These may vary according to the type of urine alarm (e.g., whether the sensor is worn in the underwear or the alarm is strapped to the wrist). The following recommendations by Kainz (2002) should be considered:

- For children who awaken at the sound of an alarm, place the alarm in a position that will require child to get out of bed to shut it off.
- Children should wear thin underwear or pajamas so that urine contacts alarm on bedsheet as quickly as possible.
- Parents/caregivers should go to their children at the sound of the alarm, but the children should shut off the alarm.
- When children do not awaken, shake them gently.
- Parents/caregivers should record bedtime, time of wetting, a rough estimate of the amount of wetting, and time of awakening next morning.
- Keep the sensor clean to avoid false alarms.
- Make sure the children are given plausible and age-appropriate explanation for bedwetting.

Research Issues

Although the behavioral treatment of enuresis has been relatively successful and the implementation of relapse prevention strategies is likely to improve its long-term effectiveness, there remain 20% to 25% of children who will not respond to these treatments. Examining physiologic/biologic factors that determine the efficacy of behavioral or medication treatments will be needed to improve the cure rate of nocturnal enuresis (Jarvelin, 2000). Both psychologic (e.g., the child's cognitive construction of enuresis; Butler, Redfern, & Forsythe, 1990) and biologic (e.g., the role of arousability from sleep) factors will need to be addressed in future studies.

8 Encopresis

Encopresis, a common problem occurring in approximately 2% to 3% of children 5 years of age, is defined as defecation in inappropriate places by children at least 4 years of age, once per month for 3 months (American Psychiatric Association, 1994). About 3% of pediatrician visits are for encopresis (Loening-Baucke, 1993). Children are also classified as having primary encopresis if they never achieved appropriate bowel control or secondary encopresis if they develop soiling following a period of fecal continence. The large majority of children with encopresis also have co-occurring constipation, making treatment even more difficult. Children often complain of abdominal pain if they are impacted. Chronic constipation can also result in significant medical problems such as megacolon, rectal bleeding, and prolapse. Fecal incontinence can also have significant effects on a child's emotional well-being and social relations (Bernard-Bonnin, Haley, Belanger, & Nadeau, 1993).

The rate of encopresis among children between 10 and 12 years of age drops to about 1% (Houts & Abramson, 1990). Nonetheless, about half of the children treated for encopresis complain of continued constipation at long-term follow-up, and many children demonstrate symptoms 3.5 to 5 years following a medical intervention (Bernard-Bonnin et al., 1993; Staiano, Andreotti, Greco, Basile, & Auricchio, 1994). McGrath, Mellon, and Murphy (2000) reviewed the literature on the treatment of encopresis for the *Journal of Pediatric Psychology*'s Empirically Supported Treatments Series. McGrath et al. identified 42 treatment studies, 13 of which were single-case designs. They classified these interventions into four categories: medical, biofeedback, psychotherapy, and behavioral interventions. However, medical interventions of some sort are used in all behavioral interventions. These typically include clean-out with laxative maintenance, dietary recommendations, and sitting schedule recommendations. In this chapter, we describe the findings with the behavioral inter-

115

ventions. First, medical interventions commonly used in these programs are described.

Using Standard Medical Interventions in Practice

Standard medical interventions are used to address the constipation and bowel impaction encountered in up to 75% of children with encopresis (Levine, 1975). Further, 57% to 86% of children present with a history of painful defecation, which also needs to be addressed (Partin, Hamill, & Fischel, 1992). The three primary interventions include cleaning out the colon, softening the bowel movements, and improving the dietary fiber intake. Recommendations vary by physician, and psychologists should tailor their program to the recommendations used by the referring physician. The intensity of medical intervention is typically determined by the findings of a thorough medical assessment. The medical examination, which will typically include rectal exam and X-ray of the abdomen, is an essential precursor to effective management of this disorder.

A common set of medical management procedures is shown in table 8.1. Other medical guidelines have been reviewed by Loening-Baucke (2002) and Pashankar, Loening-Baucke, and Bishop (2003). A typical bowel clean-out plan used at the Mayo Clinic includes one adult Fleet enema (day 1), one Dulcolax suppository (day 2), and one oral Dulcolax tablet (day 3). This 3-day cycle is repeated five times for a total of 15 days of bowel clean-out (M. Mellon, personal communication, October 12, 2003). The goal of the medical treatment is to (a) clean out the bowel and (b) allow for the child to produce at least one soft-formed bowel movement each day. The minimally necessary amount of medical treatment to achieve bowel regularity (including diet for long-term maintenance) is recommended with adjustments made over time as indicated.

Biofeedback Plus Medical Intervention

McGrath et al. (2000) identified nine studies that used biofeedback of some sort for children with encopresis. In three of the studies, the biofeedback component was designed to address the finding that many children with encopresis paradoxically contract their external anal sphincter when attempting to have a bowel movement. The medical management of these studies included bowel clean-out with laxative maintenance, fiber recommendations, and a sitting schedule. These studies also used some type of electromyographic (EMG) feedback to teach the child to relax the anal sphincter in order to defecate. Five of the studies found

Table 8.1. Parent/Caregiver Guidelines for Medical Management of Encopresis

Below are a variety of recommendations for the medical treatment of a child with encopresis. Please follow only the instructions circled by your doctor. Do not implement all recommendations.

I. Cleaning out the colon

Give a mineral oil enema followed 20 minutes later by a saline or hypotonic phosphate enema, such as a Fleet enema (do this ___ nights in a row). If there is a large result from the last enema, repeat for ____ more nights. Enemas come prepackaged. They are nonprescription and may be purchased at any supermarket or drug store.

Dulcolax suppository. Apply Vaseline to the flat end of the suppository and insert into your child's rectum, flat end first. Do this for _____ nights.

Magnesium citrate. Give ____ oz. of liquid. Do not mix it with any other liquid. Repeat in 6 hours if your child has not had a large bowel movement.

Other:

II. Softening the bowel movement

Mineral oil. Give _____ tablespoons every day. A typical starting point is 2 tablespoons in order to produce 1 to 2 soft bowel movements per day. Mineral oil can be given by spoon but is usually taken better if mixed in juice and is drunk through a straw. Keep the bottle in the refrigerator to improve the taste. Mineral oil may be bought in any supermarket or drug store. You may see some orange oil staining the underwear. This usually means that oil is leaking around hard stool in the rectum. Give your child one mineral oil and one Fleet enema. If your child has leakage or diarrhea, the dose of oil is too high. Decrease the dose by 1 teaspoon every day until the stools become firmer.

Senokot. Give ____ tablets/teaspoons every day at ____. Go up by ____ tablet/teaspoon *every day* until bowel movements are very soft and occur every day. (Granule dose: ____). Senokot will soften the bowel movement and give your child the urge to go to the bathroom within 6–8 hours. Tablets may be crushed; both tablets and liquid may be mixed in milk or applesauce. Granules should not be crushed but may be mixed in food. Senokot is nonprescription and may be found in any supermarket or drug store. Senokot is a stimulant and as such improves effectiveness of colonic and rectal muscle contractions. However, because of its stimulant properties, there is a potential for dependence to develop with long-term use.

Bulking agents (Metamucil, Citrucel, Fiberall, etc.). Give ____ tablespoons or _____ cookies/wafers every day with 8 oz. of fluid. Best taken if powder is mixed in juice. These are natural vegetable products and will soften and form up the bowel movement.

Milk of magnesia. Give _____ tablespoons every day (use half the dose if using double-strength liquid). Go up by 1 teaspoon every day until the bowel movements are very soft and occur daily.

Lactulose. Give _____ tablespoons _____ times a day. Go up by _____ tablespoons every day until the bowel movements are very soft and occur daily. Lactulose is an indigestible sugar that pulls water into the bowel movement to soften it. It is available by prescription only.

(Continued)

Table 8.1. *(Continued)*

MiraLax (polyethylene glycol powder). Mix 17 grams in 240 cc of water or juice stock; give 1.0 g/kg/day and divide doses twice daily. Titrate dose at 3-day intervals to achieve mushy stool consistency. MiraLax is available by prescription only and dissolves into the stock solution used to make it with minimal taste. MiraLax is classified as an osmotic and acts as a stool softener.

Other:

III. High-fiber diet

Your child should have at least one fiber food (minimum of 3 grams of fiber in serving) at each meal. The recommended amount of daily dietary fiber for all children is 5 grams plus your child's age in years. Some experts recommend a higher fiber amount for children recovering from functional constipation and soiling—10 grams plus your child's age in years.

Fiber without clear liquids will constipate. Make sure your child receives sufficient clear liquids (nondairy, noncaffeinated). In general, 2 ounces of nondairy fluids are recommended for each gram of fiber intake. Minimize dairy products (ice cream, cheese, milk, yogurt). Use 1% or 2% milk if your child is older than 2 years. Your child should have no more than three 8-ounce servings of dairy products per day.

Increase the amount of fruit and vegetables your child eats, at least 4–5 servings per day. Raw and crunchy fruits and vegetables are the best. Fresh is better than frozen; frozen is better than canned. Dried fruit is an excellent source of fiber.

Apple juice and bananas tend to be constipating and should be minimized. Apple cider may be substituted. Apples with the peel on are fine.

Use whole grain bread, pasta, and cereals. Examples: whole wheat, rye, bran, or oatmeal bread; Nutrigrain waffles; cereals such as Raisin Bran, Frosted Bran, Fruit 'n Fibre, Cracklin' Oat Bran, All-Bran, MultiGrain Cheerios, or Frosted Mini-Wheats. (Rice Krispies and Kix are low in fiber; sugared cereals contain no fiber.)

Encourage fruit juices and extra fluid. Pulpy juices are best (orange, tropical mixes, prune, purple grape). Juicy Juice and punch are fine. Kool-Aid and water do not contain fiber but will give extra fluid. Sodas should be avoided.

Benefiber may be added to foods or mixed into beverages to increase the fiber content. It is a natural, soluble fiber that can be mixed into food without changing the taste or texture. Benefiber provides 3 grams of fiber per tablespoon. Benefiber is sold in grocery and drug stores.

Fiber juices can be purchased and are premade to be high in fiber. These juices are sold in single-serving bottles or boxes and come in a variety of flavors. Two specific brands are Optimize (14 grams per 10 ounces; available by mail order and in stores) and Juice Plus Fibre (10 grams per 8 ounces; available by mail order only). These juices are good options for maintaining a high-fiber diet when traveling or away from home.

Crushed All-Bran may be added to food to improve the fiber content. This can be mixed in hot cereal, macaroni and cheese, meatballs or hamburger, peanut butter and jelly, pudding or ice cream, etc. Use it to bread chicken. Add when baking cookies or bread. Aim for ____ tablespoons per day.

Offer high-fiber snacks. Examples include celery and carrot sticks (plain or with peanut butter), fiber bars and trail mix, raisins or prunes, bran or whole-grain muffins, oatmeal cookies, Fig or Fruit Newtons, graham crackers, nuts, popcorn, dried fruit.

Note. The blanks in the table indicate that the exact treatment recommendations will vary based on the medical exam and the size of the child.

slight superiority for the biofeedback plus medical intervention to medical intervention alone. Subgroup analyses typically indicate that biofeedback adds to the efficacy of the treatment protocol when children have abnormal defecation dynamics (McGrath et al., 2000). At longer term follow-ups, however, superiority for biofeedback gradually disappears. For example, Nolan, Catto-Smith, Coffey, and Wells (1998) randomized 29 children, 4 to 14 years of age, with abnormal defecation dynamics to either medical treatment alone or medical treatment plus EMG biofeedback training. Four weekly biofeedback sessions were conducted. All but one of the 14 children in the biofeedback group were able to learn to relax the external anal sphincter. At 6-month follow-up, remission or improvement occurred in 29% of the biofeedback group and 40% of the medical intervention alone group. Improvement in defecation dynamics was not directly linked to a reduction in soiling. Biofeedback plus medical intervention is a probably efficacious intervention. Nolan et al. (1998) concluded that the time and expense of biofeedback training is not justified over standard medical care given the modest results of their study and other controlled studies.

Studies of Biofeedback Published Since 1998

There have been no additional studies published examining biofeedback plus medical intervention since the McGrath et al. (2000) review article. Therefore, it remains a probably efficacious intervention.

Using Biofeedback for Encopresis in Practice

Biofeedback for encopresis can be best conceptualized as retraining of the pelvic musculature. Cooperation from the patient is necessary for the procedure to be successful. A general description of a biofeedback protocol, adapted from Dahl et al. (1991) and Nolan et al. (1998), is provided here. Readers interested in using biofeedback will need to receive training from practitioners with experience and skill in implementing these protocols.

The first step in implementing a biofeedback protocol is education. Education is necessary in order for the child to understand the underlying problem and how relaxation of the external sphincter while attempting to have a bowel movement is the key to success. An explanation of the equipment is also necessary because many children and parents/caregivers will be wary of the use of equipment for this problem. EMG-monitoring equipment is available from different manufacturers with both internal and surface electrodes available.

Internal probes provide more accurate recording of sphincter activity but are also more invasive and potentially upsetting to the child. Surface electrodes are sufficient in most cases and are described here.

Surface EMG feedback of the perianal musculature is possible by placing two electrodes adjacent to the anus and a reference electrode on the thigh. A second electrode placement is also used to record abdominal muscle activity. The active electrodes are placed on both sides of the belly button with the reference electrode placed on the hip. Visual or auditory feedback from the two placements is then provided to the child. The combination of perianal and abdominal feedback allows the clinician and the child to determine if pushing or straining to have a bowel movement is done correctly (i.e., relaxing the perianal musculature while contracting the stomach muscles via a Valsalva maneuver).

In the first session, the child is asked to attempt a bowel movement so that the EMG placement can provide feedback regarding inappropriate contraction of the anal sphincter. Subsequent sessions are then used to teach the child to relax the anal sphincter while contracting the abdominal muscles. The therapist attempts to shape the appropriate response by prompting the child to squeeze the abdomen while relaxing the external sphincter. Feedback is used to determine when the response is correct. The child is asked to describe the sensation experienced when the external sphincter is relaxed. This is not always easily accomplished, but when successful it gives the child a label for this feeling of relaxing the external sphincter that can be used when having a bowel movement.

A biofeedback protocol can be implemented in a variety of ways (e.g., daily outpatient treatment over a week period or weekly sessions with home practice using a portable biofeedback device). Sphincter training programs in which the child contracts and relaxes the anal sphincter are often used. A general relaxation procedure is also often taught to the child for use just prior to attempting to defecate. The rationale for this latter procedure is that a relaxed state will result in better concentration during toileting and, in turn, a greater likelihood that the procedure for relaxing the anal sphincter will be successful.

Extensive Behavioral Intervention Plus Medical Intervention

McGrath et al. (2000) identified two interventions that combined behavioral and medical interventions in the treatment of encopresis. Stark and colleagues conducted two studies (Stark, Owens-Stively, Spirito, Lewis, & Guevremont, 1990; Stark et al., 1997) of an intervention that included an initial clean-out, dietary education with specific goals for fiber and water intake, monitoring of bowel activity, goal setting, a sitting schedule, reinforcement, and skill building. Both of these single-group interventions resulted in improvement of constipation and incontinence. In the original study (Stark, Owens-Stively, et al., 1990), 16 of 18 children (89%) were cured at the end of treatment, and 14 maintained their gains at 6-month follow-up. In the second study (Stark et al., 1997), 86% improved at the end of treatment.

Another group of studies compared full medical intervention plus behavioral intervention to full medical intervention plus behavioral intervention and biofeedback (Cox, Sutphen, Borowitz, Kovatchev, & Ling, 1998; Cox, Sutphen, Ling, Quillian, & Borowitz, 1996). These studies found that the combination of medical and behavioral interventions, with or without biofeedback, was significantly superior to medical management alone. These interventions meet the criteria for probably efficacious treatments.

Studies of Extensive Behavioral Intervention Published Since 1998

Borowitz, Cox, Sutphen, and Kovatchev (2002) provide long-term follow-up data on the Cox et al. (1998) study in which 87 children with encopresis were randomized to one of three groups: intensive medical therapy (IMT) alone, IMT plus their extended behavior management program called Enhanced Toilet Training (ETT), and IMT and ETT plus external anal sphincter biofeedback (BF). All three conditions resulted in significant improvements in daily bowel movements in the toilet, self-initiated toileting, and decreases in average daily soiling at 3-, 6-, and 12-month follow-up. At 12-month follow-up, the cure rates across the three groups (36%, 48%, and 37%) were not significantly different. The improvement rate at 12 months was significantly higher in the ETT group (78%) than for the IMT group (45%) or BF group (54%). In all three groups, response to the first 2 weeks of treatment was highly correlated with improvement at follow-up.

Because it is a long-term follow-up of an intervention study originally reviewed in McGrath et al. (2000), this study does not add to the literature on efficacy. There has been one innovative study of an extensive behavioral intervention published since 1998. Ritterband et al. (2003) randomly assigned 24 children with encopresis to either standard medical care or standard medical care plus an Internet intervention. The Internet site included more then 200 Web pages with audio that covered the components found in the ETT program (Cox et al., 1998), including education on anatomy and physiology, reinforcement for appropriate toileting, instructions and modeling in appropriate defecation dynamics, and exercises to enhance voluntary control of the external anal sphincter. The Internet site included three core modules covering anatomy, physiology, and pathophysiology of bowel movements; education on clean-outs and laxative treatments; and behavioral treatment of encopresis. Material is presented in an engaging format and includes a question-and-answer game after each core module as well as a personalized instruction sheet for each child. The three core modules require a total of 60 to 90 minutes to complete. Two weekly follow-up sessions are used to assess problems and identify any additional modules (27 are available) that need to be reviewed based on their progress. Additional modules include topics such as working with schools, taking trips, adjusting laxatives, fear of pain, and fear of toileting. The Internet site was accessed an average of 14 times by each family in the experimental group. Children in the Internet condition improved significantly more than the standard care group in terms of both accidents (one every 2 weeks vs. one accident per day) and bowel movements in the toilet. The Internet group also had a higher cure rate (70%) than did standard care (45%). This intervention seems very promising but will need to be replicated to establish its efficacy.

Using Behavioral Interventions for Encopresis in Practice

Behavioral interventions for encopresis should be preceded by education regarding encopresis. This information should have been provided by the referring physician but should be repeated by the psychologist. Education should include diagrams or drawings to assist in the explanation of "stretched-out" bowels that have lost muscle tone. The colon can be described as a pipe that is used to carry away bowel movements. Muscles are needed to expel the waste, and nerves are important in signaling the child that a bowel movement is about to occur. Children with soiling problems have "weak" muscles and nerves, which results in not emptying themselves completely or not having frequent enough bowel movements. This leads to waste accumulating in the bowels, and when this happens, it stretches the "pipe" (colon). When the pipe is stretched, the muscles get weaker and there is not enough strength to push out the bowel movements. Any new waste that is made seeps out around the waste that has "gotten stuck" in the pipe. Because the pipe is stretched out and the muscles and nerves are weak, the child does not realize the need to go to the bathroom until underwear is soiled. The various phases of the treatment protocol are then presented as a way to build up the muscles so the child can control his or her bowel movements. A sample toileting program is described in a handout designed for parents/caregivers shown in table 8.2.

Besides praising the child, parents/caregivers may also provide the child with rewards for elimination in the toilet. Spending time with parents/caregivers is an effective reinforcer for many children. Many children would rather have had 10 to 15 minutes with one of their parents/caregivers (doing such things as playing games) than tangible or material rewards. One of the advantages of using time with parents/caregivers as a reward is that it can be varied as the child desires. Regardless of what reinforcer is decided on, the child should receive the reinforcer before the end of the day. It is also important that the parents/caregivers verbally praise the child on any day that he or she does not soil. Additional time with parents/caregivers is also utilized to reward not soiling.

Table 8.2.   Parent/Caregiver Handout: Toileting Program

1. Maintain a positive approach to the problem.

2. Instruct your child to try to have a bowel movement after meals and after school. Have him or her sit for 5 to 10 minutes. Make this as pleasant as possible, but avoid distractions such as hand-held video games. Don't nag.

What to do when proper elimination has occurred:
   1. Your child should be instructed to tell you when appropriate toileting has occurred. Check the toilet for stool before the child flushes the toilet.

   2. Consistently praise your child (this is very important).

   3. Make sure your child knows how to wipe properly and is wiping with toilet paper after each bowel movement.

Monitoring:
   1. Check your child's pants frequently (at least three times per day). Be tactful so as not to embarrass your child when doing so. Keep a record of bowel movements and accidents. Verbally praise not soiling. Consider setting up a reward program.

   2. It is important that you catch soiled pants as soon as possible after the soiling has occurred. Keep an accurate count of underpants to prevent children from hiding accidents.

What to do when you child soils his or her pants:
   1. After soiling has occurred, instruct your child to:
      a. Rinse and wash out his or her own underwear and pants.
      b. Bathe quickly (just enough time to clean himself or herself). Use a bathtub with only one or two inches of water in it.
      c. Put on clean clothes.

   2. Use only enough verbal prompts to keep him or her going—no nagging. Handle soiling in a matter-of-fact manner. Do not mention the soiling episode *during or after* any of these procedures.

Praise and rewards are very important because using the toilet and proper elimination often prove quite difficult for children with soiling problems. It is important to change toileting behaviors in addition to treating underlying medical problems, so these procedures are necessary for a period of time. Often there is significant conflict and frustration between the child and parent/caregiver. "Demystifying" the problem of encopresis is important to improve family member "buy-in" and reduce blame and anger. Behavioral approaches should focus on adherence to program (i.e., those behaviors the child has control over) and not on what the child may not be able to control (i.e., accidents). Mild punishment (e.g., response-cost procedures) may be used sparingly to address nonadherence–the behaviors the child can choose to control or not control.

A number of suggestions for improving the toileting program may also be useful:

1. After the child is cleaned out and starts on a behavioral program, keep track of the length of time that expires before he or she begins to have renewed soiling incidents. These children may have a certain time cycle before they are backed up again, and you should be aware of this when devising the program.

2. For most children, the reward system will initially be used simply for attempting to have a bowel movement by sitting on the toilet. Over time, as the reward system evolves, rewards can be restricted to either attempting to go to the bathroom on his or her own without prompting, or actually having a bowel movement.

3. Many children with encopresis, it seems, do not mind cleaning up after themselves. Thus, as the program becomes more refined over time, you may need to add an overcorrection component to the cleanup, such as scrubbing the toilet bowl or washing the bathroom floor.

4. Typically, enemas are inserted by the parents/caregivers. However, depending on the age of the child, it may be appropriate for the child to eventually learn how to insert the enema after supervised practice. This behavior can be gradually shaped with comfort and support provided by parents/caregivers. The child can be reinforced for such efforts and self-control.

5. A systematic reward program is important to institute, particularly given the extended periods of time needed to successfully treat encopresis. A menu of rewards is useful because it can be modified

over time to both increase time to receiving a reward and add new rewards to generate enthusiasm.

6. You will typically be working with one parent/caregiver when treating children with encopresis. It is important to enlist other family members in the protocol given the burden of implementing the program. For example, using another family member as a reinforcer and a coach may well be an important treatment variable and should be considered whenever possible.

7. When first starting a program, ask the parents/caregivers if they observe the child actually pushing hard and attempting to have a bowel movement. It is very common for a child to sit on the toilet for 5 minutes but not really push in an attempt to have a bowel movement. If a child does not push very much on the toilet, it may reflect a motivational deficit or fear of pain. Fear of pain can be addressed by having the child first push hard after taking a suppository so that he or she can see some success without resulting in much pain.

8. It is important to explain to the parents/caregivers that successful treatment takes time and that there may be a number of ups and downs over the course of the treatment before the soiling difficulties are controlled. Estimating 6 to 12 months of treatment time for the difficult cases sets a time parameter that may help ensure cooperation for the entire program.

9. Some children may be able to report the sensations, comfortable and uncomfortable, that are associated with defecation—before, during, and after the bowel movement. Specific sensations that the child reports consistently preceding defecation may be used to help cue the child to a bowel movement. Cue rehearsal—several times daily for a few weeks—may increase the probability that a child will use the cues effectively.

10. Skill building may be necessary at the beginning of each program (i.e., children may need to practice toileting). Make sure the child knows the proper sitting position on the toilet (i.e., feet firmly on flat surface, with knees at same level as hips). Step stools can be used to make sure that the child's knees are at the correct height.

11. Goal setting should also be individually tailored to the child. Goals may include a gradual increase in toilet sitting and a gradual decrease in soiling accidents.

Positive Reinforcement and Medical Intervention

McGrath et al. (2000) identified three studies that added a positive reinforcement component to a medical intervention. Treatment in these studies consisted of a bowel clean-out followed by laxative maintenance, dietary fiber recommendations, and a sitting schedule. The open trial study (Loening-Baucke, 1989) found that almost half the children improved. One between-groups study found the intervention superior to medical treatment alone, although the medical treatment did not include clean-out and laxative therapy (Nolan, Debelle, Oberklaid, & Coffey, 1991). This intervention meets criteria for a probably efficacious intervention.

Positive Reinforcement and Medical Intervention
Without Fiber Recommendations

McGrath et al. (2000) reviewed four medical interventions with positive reinforcement but without recommendations for fiber intake. The only between-groups study (Wald, Chandra, Gabel, & Chiponis, 1987) found such an intervention to be superior to the same medical intervention plus biofeedback: 71% versus 40% cured. The other three studies were single-group designs without a comparison group, with one reporting a 75% cure rate at 1 year follow-up (Young, 1973). This intervention meets criteria for a probably efficacious intervention.

Studies of Positive Reinforcement and Medical Intervention
Published Since 1998

There have been no additional studies since 1998 of positive reinforcement and medical intervention, with or without dietary fiber recommendations. These interventions therefore remain probably efficacious.

Clinical Issues

The literature on biofeedback training is somewhat difficult to synthesize due to the diverse underlying presentations of children in most studies. Patients in these studies may have constipation, incontinence, or constipation plus incontinence. Many have physiologically determined abnormal defecation dynamics (e.g., Loening-Baucke, 1990).

Broadly stated, it appears that adding a behavioral intervention to a medical intervention improves outcomes in children without abnormal defecation dynamics. Biofeedback may increase the efficacy of treatment outcomes for children with abnormal defecation dynamics. However, more recent studies question whether biofeedback is of added value. Gains in treatment with biofeedback rarely occur after 6 months, suggesting that a different or more intensive intervention should be considered at this point if symptoms persist (McGrath et al., 2000). Group interventions have been tested and look promising, in terms of not only their efficacy but also cost-effectiveness.

Although one parent/caregiver will most often come to treatment sessions and take primary responsibility for the program, the key to a successful program is to involve other caregivers in the home in the treatment protocol. Other family members might include grandparents/caregivers or other adult family members living in the home. Sometimes other adult family members may undermine the program, and it is important to ensure that the caregiver implementing the program can manage any such interference in the household.

Research Issues

McGrath et al. (2000) note a number of important issues that need to be considered in future research. Studies vary widely in their reports of success, at least partly due to reporting different outcome criteria (e.g., fewer accidents, cure rates, etc.). This methodological weakness in the literature makes it difficult to conclude that any one of these interventions is superior to another. The diagnostic heterogeneity of children with encopresis also makes it difficult to determine differential efficacy. At a minimum, descriptions of research participants should include whether they have incontinence, constipation, constipation and incontinence, or abnormal defecation dynamics. Finally, given the extensive nature of most interventions and the demands on parents/caregivers and child, adherence to the regimen needs to be systematically assessed in future studies.

9 Sleep Problems in Young Children

Bedtime difficulties and frequent night wakings are experienced by about one-quarter of children between 1 and 5 years of age and are one of the most common complaints presented by parents/caregivers to pediatricians (Mindell, Moline, Zendell, Brown, & Fry, 1994). These sleep disturbances also tend to persist. For example, Kataria, Swanson, and Trevathan (1987) found that 84% of their sample of children had persistent sleep problems after 3 years. In a long-term, longitudinal study, sleep problems were found to be more likely at both 5 and 10 years of age in those children who had sleep problems before the age of 6 months (Pollock, 1992, 1994).

For children with sleep problems, falling asleep is often associated with any number of parental maneuvers, such as lying down with the child. The child, in turn, may have difficulty sleeping unless those conditions are in place. Psychosocial interventions are therefore often recommended based on the frequent observation that parents/caregivers play an important role in maintaining bedtime difficulties and night wakings. These types of problems naturally lend themselves to behavioral treatment approaches. Indeed, almost all published nonmedical treatment studies for early childhood sleep problems have utilized behavioral strategies.

Mindell (1999) provided a comprehensive review of the literature on bedtime problems (e.g., bedtime refusal, bedtime tantrums) and frequent night wakings as part of the *Journal of Pediatric Psychology*'s Empirically Supported Treatments Series. Only studies with children 5 years old and younger were included. A total of 41 studies were evaluated. Parental education and early preventive intervention for parents/caregivers of infants have also been shown to be effective in reducing sleep onset and night waking (Kuhn & Elliott, 2003; Meltzer & Mindell, 2004) but are not reviewed here. Four specific behavioral interventions were identified as occurring most frequently in the Mindell review: extinction, graduated extinction, positive routines, and scheduled awakenings. A fifth group of studies, using different packages of interventions, primarily as multicomponent treatment programs, was also evaluated. Below the findings of the Mindell review are summarized, broken down by treatment technique. The reader is referred to the Mindell (1999) article for more details. A recent article by Kuhn and Elliott (2003) also reviews behavioral interventions for both bedtime refusal and night wakings, as well as circadian rhythm disorders and parasomnias. At the end of each section below are included any additional treatment articles that have been published since the Mindell (1999) review.

Extinction

When used in reference to sleep problems, the term *extinction* refers to a procedure whereby the parents/caregivers put a child to bed at a certain bedtime and then systematically ignore any whining or crying by the child until a set wake-up time the next morning. In some procedures, parents/caregivers are instructed to check on the child's safety in as nonreinforcing a manner as possible.

Three separate research groups have demonstrated the effectiveness of extinction for sleep problems in well-controlled, between-subject, randomized studies. One study demonstrated the superiority of extinction to scheduled awakenings (Rickert & Johnson, 1988). France (1992; France, Blampied, & Wilkinson, 1991) showed extinction to be effective, especially when combined with medication (trimeprazine). Seymour, Bayfield, Brock, and During (1983) demonstrated the effectiveness of extinction in conjunction with a set bedtime routine using a within-subjects design. In a randomized trial, Seymour, Brock, During, and Poole (1989) demonstrated that extinction, whether implemented with therapist support or via parent psychoeducation, was superior to a wait-list control condition.

Two other studies have also evaluated extinction for sleep problems with somewhat modified procedures. Chadez and Nurius (1987) treated a 7-month-old with extinction, but had to first address parental concerns about the procedure by better describing the rationale for the treatment as well as the parents' concerns about the potential negative effects on their infant. Rapoff, Christophersen, and Rapoff (1982) trained nurse practitioners who then treated six children with sleep problems by using a set bedtime and bedtime routine and then extinction. If the child came out of the bedroom, the parents/caregivers administered one spank and, without talking, returned the child to his or her bed. Parents/caregivers were given all instructions in writing and encouraged to call the nurse practitioner if they had problems or questions. They were also given instructions on how to administer the spank in a calm, controlled manner. One parent questioned the necessity of the spank and decided to return the child to bed without spanking but also without attention or talking. The procedure was effective for half the families. The authors concluded that parents/caregivers in this primary care intervention need continued support during the intervention. Taken as a whole, these studies support extinction as a well-established intervention.

Studies of Extinction Published Since 1998

Since the publication of the Mindell (1999) review article, one study was conducted comparing extinction to graduated extinction (described below). Reid, Walter, and O'Leary (1999) randomized 49 toddlers to standard extinction, graduated extinction, or a wait-list condition. Both of the extinction conditions resulted in improved bedtime behavior and fewer nighttime sleep problems. Some families had difficulties with the procedure and dropped out of treatment. Mothers in the graduated extinction condition reported higher rates of compliance and lower treatment-related distress than did mothers in the extinction condition. Mothers in the graduated extinction group also reported improvements in the parent–child relationship.

Using Extinction in Practice

Extinction is a difficult procedure to implement. Therefore, it is important for clinicians to adequately prepare parents/caregivers for using extinction. Parents/caregivers should be made aware of how difficult it is to ignore their child's crying. Each child is being taught a new skill—to self-soothe—and parents/caregivers should be reminded that teaching a new skill takes practice and time. The time to successful implementation of extinction typically ranges from 2 weeks to 1 month, if parents/caregivers are consistent and don't provide intermittent reinforcement for crying (e.g., by occasionally rocking their child or bringing their child into bed with them).

Given the difficulty of implementing extinction, parents/caregivers should be warned not to start the procedure under times of high family stress. In families with two adult caregivers, whatever the combination (two parents, one parent and a grandparent, etc.), both family members should ideally be actively involved and support each other. In single-parent families, these procedures are typically very difficult. Some single parents enlist the help of a friend or relative; sometimes, for example, a close relative sleeps over for 1 to 2 weeks to assist the parent in program implementation. Other setting factors should be considered, such as making the child's crib and bedroom as inviting and comfortable as possible and introducing a transitional/love object for young children who might not have one. Stuffed animals and blankets help children feel secure when parents/caregivers aren't available. A set bedtime and bedtime routine should already have been established. Extinction is facilitated when the child is drowsy, but awake, when put to bed. Parents/caregivers need to be instructed about extinction bursts—escalation of the intensity of the problem behavior—to counteract any beliefs that implementing the procedure is only worsening the problem. They should also be aware that extinction bursts are more likely to occur with extinction procedures than with graduated extinction or parental presence (Lawton, France, & Blampied, 1991).

Extinction procedures often fail when therapists are inflexible in their implementation. Therapists must be cognizant of the fact that extinction is a difficult concept to accept as a parent, is often foreign to the belief systems of parents, and is at odds with natural parenting instincts. Thus, it is important to establish a strong working alliance with parents and to modify the technique so that it fits within the family mores and structure. Graduated extinction, described below, is often more acceptable to parents.

Graduated Extinction

Many parents/caregivers find it very difficult to ignore a young child's crying long enough for extinction to be effective. For those parents/caregivers not willing to have their child "cry it out" for extended periods, the use of a graduated extinction procedure has been advocated. Mindell (1999) reported on one well-controlled, randomized study and a number of within-subject and multiple-baseline studies using graduated extinction.

L. A. Adams and Rickert (1989) instructed parents/caregivers to ignore bedtime tantrums for specific periods of time based on the child's age and the amount of time that the parents/caregivers believed that they could ignore their child. Each week, the length of time parents/caregivers waited to comfort the child was increased. At the designated time, the parents/caregivers comforted their tantrumming child for 15 seconds or less. If the child left the bedroom, the parents/caregivers returned the child to the bedroom and the child was firmly told to return to sleep. This procedure was effective in reducing number and intensity of tantrums compared to a control group, but a less aversive procedure, positive routines, was equally as effective.

Other studies have shown graduated extinction to be useful but not better than other treatments. For example, Sadeh (1994) randomly assigned 50 infants to a graduated extinction treatment or co-sleeping, in which one of the parents/caregivers slept in the child's bedroom for 1 week without having any other involvement with the child during the night. Results indicted that more than half of the children significantly improved, but there was no difference between the two interventions.

Several multiple baseline studies have also been reported. Lawton et al. (1991) treated seven children with night wakings using graduated extinction in a multiple-baseline design. First, an individually set time that each parent paid attention to their child at bedtime was established. Parents/caregivers then reduced this attending time by one-seventh every 4 days so that by 28 days there was no parental attention given to the child. Following the first 28 days, the parents/caregivers were told not to attend to their child between bedtime and morning wake time, unless it was deemed absolutely necessary. This procedure successfully reduced the frequency and duration of night wakings in half the children. A fourth child had a significant reduction in the duration of night wakings.

Mindell and Durand (Durand & Mindell, 1990; Mindell & Durand, 1993) asked parents/caregivers to wait progressively longer periods of time, in 5-minute increments, before checking on their child during a night waking. Each subsequent night, the time was increased by 5 minutes, with the longest period being 20 minutes. In the first study, night wakings were successfully treated first in a 14-month-old child. Problems with settling at bedtime also eventually resolved. In the second study (Mindell & Durand, 1993), six children were treated for bedtime problems before night wakings in a multiple-baseline across-subjects design. Successful treatment of bedtime problems generalized to night wakings for five of the six subjects. This study suggests that when children can learn to fall asleep on their own, subsequent night wakings may also resolve. Based on these studies, graduated extinction can be considered a probably efficacious intervention.

Studies of Graduated Extinction Published Since 1998

Since the publication of the Mindell (1999) review article, the Reid et al. (1999) study, described above, compared extinction to graduated extinction. There were no differences between conditions. No other studies have been reported. Thus, graduated extinction remains a probably efficacious intervention.

Using Graduated Extinction in Practice

Although easier to implement than extinction, graduated extinction still involves a great deal of patience and effort on the part of the parents/caregivers. Meltzer and Mindell (2004) note that there are four different areas in which the clinician can tailor graduated extinction: the amount of physical contact between parent/caregiver and child, the proximity of parent/caregiver to child (in room, out of room), duration of time between checks, and duration of check itself. All the comments made above in the section on extinction—preparing the parents/caregivers, being consistent, and establishing the best setting factors—apply to graduated extinction. After completing the bedtime routine (e.g., a bath and a story), the child should be placed in the bed or crib and parents/caregivers should be instructed to leave the room. At bedtime or during the night, if the child is yelling, calling out, or lightly crying, but remains in bed, parents/caregivers should be instructed to respond once to the child that it is bedtime and they will not answer any further calls. If the child begins to cry more, table 9.1 presents a typical progression for gradually increasing time periods before checking on the child (Ferber, 1985).

Table 9.1.   Number of Minutes to Wait Before Checking on Your Crying Child

	First check	Second check	Third and all other checks
Day 1	5	10	15
Day 2	10	15	20
Day 3	15	20	25
Day 4	20	25	30
Day 5	25	30	35

Note. Adapted with the permission of Simon & Schuster Adult Publishing Group from *How to Solve Your Child's Sleep Problems,* by R. Ferber, 1985, p. 78, New York: Simon & Schuster. Copyright 1985 by Richard Ferber.

Checks can be progressively longer within one night or across successful nights. Checking on the child should be brief, one minute at maximum, reassuring but with minimal interaction and talk. Patting on the back is permissible but the visit should be boring for the child, not too reinforcing, and not include picking up the child or lying down with the child. This procedure is designed to reassure the child that the parents/caregivers are still present and to reassure the parent/caregiver that their child is okay. The checking is not designed to help the child fall asleep—the premise behind the procedure is that the child needs to fall asleep on his or her own. "Quick checks"—checks that occur at consistent intervals, such as 10 minutes—may be comparably effective (Pritchard & Appleton, 1988) and easier for some parents/caregivers to implement.

If the child gets out of bed, comes out of the bedroom, or comes into the parents/caregivers' room, parents/caregivers should be instructed to be firm and return the child to bed. It is very important to return the child to bed every time he or she gets up. This is often the most difficult part of the program, because parents/caregivers are understandably exhausted and frustrated in the middle of the night.

If the child continues to get out of bed, parents/caregivers should inform the child that they will close the bedroom door if the child gets up again. If the child gets back out of bed, parents/caregivers should be instructed to put the child back in bed and close the door for 1 minute. After the time is up, open the door. If the child is in bed, parents/caregivers should praise the child and leave the door open. If the child is up, parents/caregivers should put the child back in bed and close the door again. Parents/caregivers are typically instructed to begin a program of closing the bedroom door for gradually increasing amounts of time. Ferber (1985) suggests the schedule shown in table 9.2.

Table 9.2. Number of Minutes to Keep the Door Closed If Child Gets Out of Bed

	First closing	Second closing	Third closing	All other closings
Day 1	1	2	3	5
Day 2	2	4	6	8
Day 3	3	5	7	10
Day 4	5	7	10	15

Note. Adapted with the permission of Simon & Schuster Adult Publishing Group from *How to Solve Your Child's Sleep Problems,* by R. Ferber, 1985, p. 79, New York: Simon & Schuster. Copyright 1985 by Richard Ferber.

Parents/caregivers should be advised not to lock the child in the bedroom, but they can hold the door closed if the child is trying to open it. Parents/caregivers should also be made aware that checking may reinforce crying by virtue of parental presence.

Kuhn and Elliott (2003) also describe a procedure called *extinction with parental presence*. This intervention is based on the assumption that bedtime refusal for some children is related to separation anxiety. In this procedure, parents/caregivers sleep in the child's bedroom, either on the floor or on a cot, not in the child's bed, for 1 week. The parent/caregiver pretends to be sleeping and ignores the child. This procedure was one of the comparison conditions in the Sadeh (1994) study which was shown to be effective.

Scheduled Awakenings

Scheduled awakenings are best suited for children who experience frequent night wakings that occur at fairly regular times of the night. In scheduled awakenings, parents/caregivers wake the child approximately 15 minutes before the time the child's spontaneous night waking typically occurs. Scheduled awakenings are then faded out. A brief awakening and return to sleep is believed to forestall the child from reaching a higher level of arousal and full awakening if allowed to awaken on his or her own. This technique was originally devised for sleep walking and night terrors. Although several case reports have been published, only one randomized study (Rickert & Johnson, 1988) has examined scheduled awakenings. In a sample of 33 children with night wakings, scheduled awakening was found to be more effective than a control group and equally effective as systematic ignoring, although it took longer to achieve the desired results. Several other single-case studies with positive findings have also been reported (e.g., Johnson, Bradley-Johnson, & Stack, 1981). Thus, scheduled awakening is a probably efficacious intervention.

Studies of Scheduled Awakening Published Since 1998

No studies using scheduled awakenings for nocturnal waking have been published since the Mindell (1999) review article. Scheduled awakening remains a "probably efficacious" intervention.

Using Scheduled Awakenings in Practice

Scheduled awakenings are relatively easy to describe but often difficult to imple-ment. First, parents/caregivers must be convinced of the rationale for awaken-ing a sleeping child. Parents/caregivers often believe that the procedure will result in the child being awake for a substantial amount of time which will dis-rupt sleep even more than the presenting problem. The procedure should be used for about a month and then gradually tapered. Sleep cycles should be explained to the parents/caregivers in order for them to understand how some children move without incident to the next sleep cycle, and some become fully aroused but return to sleep with relative ease.

In the scheduled awakening procedure, parents/caregivers are asked to awaken the child 15 to 30 minutes prior to the usual time of waking, which has been determined previously with a monitoring procedure for a period of 10 days. Parents/caregivers should be instructed to awaken the child by light shaking. As the child arouses, parents/caregivers should ask the child to sit up in bed and open his or her eyes. Parents/caregivers should speak with the child and ask a few questions, with the goal being to get a simple, mumbled response. The amount of time a child should be drowsily awake in this procedure has not been studied. This will require some experimentation by the parents/caregivers with the goal being to use as short a time period as necessary to reduce the num-ber of later arousals but still enabling the child to fall back to sleep relatively eas-ily. One minute should be the maximum and 20 to 30 seconds will usually suffice.

Positive Routines

In positive routines, parents/caregivers establish a bedtime routine of calm, pleasant activities for the child. Three studies using positive bedtime routines were reviewed by Mindell (1999). Two used within-subject designs without con-trol groups and are not reviewed here. One large well-controlled study has found this technique to be effective. L. A. Adams and Rickert (1989) had parents/caregivers delay the children's bedtime to a naturally occurring later bedtime. Children engaged in four to seven enjoyable activities prior to bedtime. If a tantrum or misbehavior occurred, the child was sent to bed. After the routine was established, the parents/caregivers gradually moved the child's bedtime earlier until it coincided with the desired bedtime. Positive routines were found to be comparable to graduated extinction in effectiveness and more effective than a control group. Parents/caregivers in the positive routines group, however, reported greater marital satisfaction suggesting that this procedure may have added benefits to the parents/caregivers and family. Nonetheless, positive routines currently meet only criteria for a probably efficacious intervention.

Piazza and colleagues have also published several within-subject studies of a variation on positive routines (Piazza & Fisher, 1991; Piazza, Fisher, & Sherer, 1997). Piazza starts with a "faded bedtime," delaying bedtime by about a half hour. If the child does not fall asleep within 30 minutes of being placed in bed, the child is taken out of bed and kept awake for up to an hour. This procedure is used until the child falls asleep quickly. Once this is achieved, the bedtime is gradually set earlier in the evening until the desired bedtime is achieved. In addition to the bedtime routine, the child must be awakened at a set time each day regardless of how much he or she has slept the night before and napping not allowed. Although this variation of positive routines appears to be a useful approach, it will need to be tested by other investigators in order to become established as an effective treatment.

Studies of Positive Routines Published Since 1998

No studies examining positive routines have been published since the Mindell (1999) review.

Using Positive Routines in Practice

Positive routines should be described to parents/caregivers as a less aversive procedure for parents/caregivers and child but one that will likely take longer to implement than extinction procedures. Parents/caregivers are first asked to determine when their child would naturally fall asleep if parents/caregivers did not set a bedtime. Parents/caregivers are then asked to select four to seven quiet activities lasting in total from 20 to 30 minutes. Parents/caregivers typically start with a bath to calm the child, then move to one of the calming activities. It is preferable to engage in these quiet activities in a dimly lit room without other distractions, such as the television. Some parents/caregivers put on bedclothes to help reinforce the notion of bedtime for the entire household. Parents/caregivers should praise the child after calmly engaging in each activity. Each week the start time for the calming routines is 10 minutes earlier until the desired bedtime is reached.

Clinical Issues

There are a number of individual and family factors that will affect the efficacy of any of the treatment techniques described in this chapter. For example, children with difficult temperaments make implementing the extinction procedures particularly challenging. Family factors are also very important. For example, family living arrangements, such as a small apartment where the rooms are contiguous or the baby's crib is in the parents/caregivers' room, make using extinction difficult. The presence of extended family in the home, such as grandparents, also often makes it harder to implement these programs. For example, there can be intergenerational conflict when parents and grandparents do not agree on the use of an intervention such as extinction. Sibling issues will also affect implementation of behavioral plans (e.g., when siblings share a room or a sibling is easily awakened during the night). Parental exhaustion and sleep deprivation are important to consider when determining the best time to implement these procedures.

Any underlying caregiver issue, such as anxiety, depression, or marital conflict, or family issue, such as stressors related to financial difficulties or major life events like a job change, has the potential to disrupt the program. Successful implementation of these interventions may affect the caregivers in a positive fashion. For example, one study demonstrated that a successful intervention improved maternal depressive symptoms (Hiscock & Wake, 2002). Parents/caregivers are particularly prone to intermittent reinforcement of negative behaviors that interfere with the behavioral program when the factors described above are operating. For example, it is common for tired parents/caregivers to "give in" and let their child engage in a sleep behavior (e.g., sleeping in the parental bed), especially when implementing extinction procedures. This lapse in following the behavioral guidelines will result in a longer time to improved behavior or failure of the program. Thus, these background family issues must be addressed in the context of the behavioral program.

A second important clinical issue is treatment acceptability and compliance. Typically, the least acceptable option for parents/caregivers often results in poor parental adherence. Rickert and Johnson (1988) note that 10% of the families in their study refused to participate once they learned they were assigned to the extinction condition. In addition, a number of parents/caregivers had originally refused to consent to the study when they were informed their child might be assigned to the extinction condition. Most parents/caregivers who refuse to use extinction cite concerns about the possible negative effects on emotional development. Graduated extinction, which has less research support than extinction, is a much more acceptable approach to most parents/caregivers. Parental compliance with scheduled awakenings may prove difficult either because parents/caregivers are skeptical of the wisdom of waking a sleeping child or the parents/caregivers dislike or have difficulty awakening themselves during the night to institute treatment (Johnson et al., 1981; Johnson & Lerner, 1985).

Finally, the origin of sleep problems will affect the clinician's choice of treatment techniques and needs to be considered. For example, a behavioral approach alone may be useful for a child with poor sleep associations. However, other therapeutic strategies will need to be incorporated when a child's sleep problems are related to parent-child difficulties.

Research Issues

There are a number of methodological problems in existing studies which will need to be addressed in the next generation of research. First, the reliance on parent report to evaluate outcome raises concerns. The validity of parental sleep diaries has been called into question even though the few studies that have used objective measures, such as videotape or audiotape, to evaluate sleep diaries provide support for the validity of parental report (e.g., France & Hudson, 1990; Mindell & Durand, 1993; Rapoff et al., 1982). Actigraphy devices, sensors worn on the wrist that allow continuous monitoring of motion to determine sleep–wake patterns, have also been used for validation purposes. When actigraphy measures are used (e.g., Sadeh, 1994), discrepancies between this objective measure and parental diaries are noted. That is, many children with sleep problems continued to awaken at night after treatment but fell back to sleep on their own. Parents/caregivers may also record fewer awakenings the longer they are asked to complete sleep logs (Sadeh, 1996).

Length of follow-up is another methodological weakness in the literature. A follow-up period of several weeks to 6 months is common. Successfully treated sleep problems are often quiescent for relatively long periods of time but then may return during childhood. Thus, longer follow-up studies are needed to guide future clinical work. In addition, many sleep problems persist, at varying levels of intensity, sometimes into adolescence.

The usefulness of differential treatment approaches for sleep problems which arise from different etiologies has yet to be investigated (Minde, 1999). The differing etiologies of bedtime tantrums, for example, are clearly taken into consideration by clinicians when conducting a functional analysis of the problem behavior and selecting the appropriate behavioral techniques, even if the research literature has not clearly delineated which strategies are best (K. Brown & Piazza, 1999).

Most research to date has combined samples of children who have bedtime problems only, those who have night wakings only, and those with both types of sleep problems. Studies with more homogeneous samples may assist clinicians in devising more targeted interventions. Finally, the efficacy of specific individual components within multicomponent treatment packages has yet to be determined. Although many of the components of these packages are easily delivered and do not create additional burdens for clinicians, dismantling research will help us determine the most parsimonious treatment approach. Such studies should also determine the treatments most acceptable to parents/caregivers and the simplest to implement.

PROMISING INTERVENTIONS FOR SPECIFIC DISORDERS

10 Cystic Fibrosis

Cystic fibrosis (CF) is a genetically inherited disease that affects approximately 30,000 persons in the United States (Cystic Fibrosis Foundation, 2003). CF affects the secretory glands of major organs in the respiratory, gastrointestinal, and reproductive systems. Pancreatic insufficiency and chronic progressive pulmonary disease result from the underlying defect and eventually lead to premature death due typically to cardiorespiratory failure. Medical advances have resulted in prolonged life expectancies over the last two decades, with the mean life expectancy currently 32.2 years (Cystic Fibrosis Foundation, 2003). These new treatments have resulted in a very demanding medical regimen. Optimal adherence is important to survival but places significant stress on both patients and their families.

Treatment of CF includes a demanding regimen of chest physiotherapy; antibiotics, pancreatic replacement enzymes, and fat-soluble vitamins; and consumption of 120% to 150% of the recommended daily dietary allowance. This latter recommendation helps offset the energy loss from malabsorption and the higher energy demands resulting from lung disease. Studies on adherence to the medical regimen suggest that patients with CF have particular difficulties adhering to their chest physiotherapy and dietary regimens. In view of this demanding regimen, behavioral interventions to improve adherence are indicated.

Interventions to Improve Adherence to Single Components of the CF Medical Regimen

The *Journal of Pediatric Psychology*'s Empirically Supported Treatment Series did not review the literature on interventions to improve adherence to the medical regimen in patients with CF. However, there is a limited literature on interventions with this population that have typically targeted specific components of the medical regimen (e.g., chest physiotherapy, exercise, and diet). These studies are reviewed below.

Chest Physiotherapy

There have been two studies examining adherence to chest physiotherapy in patients with CF. Both of these reports are single-case studies (Hagopian & Thompson, 1999; Stark, Miller, Plienes, & Drabman, 1987). Both used behavioral approaches to increase adherence, and one of the patients had mental retardation and autism in addition to CF. Given the limited generalizability of a literature with two patients, these studies are not reviewed here.

Exercise

There have been three studies on home-based exercise reported in the literature (deJong, Grevink, Roorda, Kaptein, & van der Schans, 1994; Holzer, Schnall, & Landau, 1984; Schneiderman-Walker et al., 2000). Only the Schneiderman-Walker et al. (2000) study provided a measure of adherence to treatment, and none of these studies provided much detail regarding the interventions used to improve adherence to exercise. In the deJong et al. (1994) study, 10 adolescent patients with CF participated in home exercise training for 3 months. The exercise regimen consisted of 15 minutes of cycle training at a submaximal workload each day. Twice per week this exercise regimen was supervised by a physiotherapist. After the 3-month supervised trial, patients were asked to continue cycling at home for an additional month without physiotherapist supervision. Significant improvement from baseline was noted on maximal exercise capacity and maximal oxygen intake. This improvement was maintained after the 1 month of exercising without supervision.

Holzer et al. (1984) assessed chest symptoms, medication usage, and physical activity of 86 children with CF. After baseline assessment, 45 children served as controls and were asked to continue with their typical level of physical activity for 3 months. The experimental group of 41 children were asked to perform a series of home exercises, primarily jogging, for 30 minutes each day for 3 months. They also participated in supervised gymnastic sessions four times over 3 months. Adherence to training was not assessed. Follow-up assessment did not indicate any differences between groups on pulmonary function data.

Schneiderman-Walker et al. (2000) randomized 72 patients with CF, between the ages of 7 and 19 years, to an exercise condition or usual physical activity control condition. In the experimental condition, exercise physiologists instructed patients on the minimum requirements of aerobic activity such as cycling, running, and swimming. Patients were instructed to engage in one of these activities for 20 minutes at least three times per week. Patients in the experimental group were also taught to monitor their heart rate, and a target heart rate was set for each patient. Patients in both groups were contacted every 4 to 6 weeks throughout the study. Compliance with the exercise regimen was rated by physiotherapists, and the average rating suggested the experimental group was partially compliant with the exercise regimen. At 3-year follow-up, the pulmonary function status of the experimental group declined more slowly than did that of the control group. Based on these three studies, behavioral interventions to increase exercise in patients with CF is a promising intervention.

Diet

Research to date has been so limited that behavioral interventions to improve adherence to chest physiotherapy and exercise cannot be classified as promising. One research team has conducted four studies examining behavioral interventions to increase caloric intake among children with CF (Stark, Bowen, Tyc, Evans, & Passero, 1990; Stark et al., 1993, 1996, 2003). This body of work results in this behavioral protocol being considered a promising intervention. The original study (Stark, Bowen, et al., 1990) tested the efficacy of a group behavioral intervention in five mildly undernourished children with CF ranging in age from 6 to 12 years. The children and their parents each participated in six outpatient group sessions. Parent and child groups were held separately. The effects of the intervention were evaluated using a multiple-baseline design in which different meals (i.e., snacks, breakfast, lunch, and dinner were targeted sequentially). The behavioral intervention consisted of nutrition education and contingency management for achieving caloric goals. Parents received information regarding the nutritional content of the meal being targeted as well as behavior management instructions on how to help children eat the foods presented. Nutrition information was individualized by providing parents with data on their child's caloric intake as calculated from diet diaries. In the children's group, children received information on how to make higher caloric food choices. Behavioral practice was also used in sessions by having children eat a meal. In addition, a reinforcement program was used wherein children earned a reward for meeting weekly home caloric goals. This single-group pretest–posttest design revealed a 25% to 43% increase in caloric intake as well as increases in weight. These treatment gains in caloric intake were maintained at 9-month follow-up.

The second study (Stark et al., 1993) essentially replicated the first study. A single-group pretest–posttest design was used with three children ranging in age from 3 to 8 years. Nutritional education plus contingency management was used to increase caloric consumption with parents and children seen in separate but simultaneous groups. This seven-session outpatient treatment used a multiple-baseline design targeting different meals sequentially as in the original study. The nutrition education and contingency management procedures were comparable to those used in the original intervention (Stark, Bowen, et al., 1990). In addition, the children were taught a relaxation exercise to help with complaints of stomach pain after meals. All three children increased caloric intake across meals, and at posttreatment total caloric intake had increased 32% to 60%. This increased consumption was maintained at a 2-year follow-up. Rates of weight and height gain were greater in the 2 years following the intervention than in the year prior to the intervention.

The third study (Stark et al., 1996) was a randomized control group study using the same behavioral intervention used in the Stark et al. (1993) study. The children in the intervention ($N = 5$) ranged in age from 5 to 10 years and were compared to a group placed in a wait-list control condition ($N = 4$). The intervention group increased their caloric intake 1,032 calories per day, while the control group increased only 244 calories per day pre- to posttreatment. The intervention group also gained significantly more weight than the control group over the 6 weeks of treatment. One month posttreatment, the intervention was conducted with two of the four children from the wait-list control group. Improved caloric intake and weight gain pre- to posttreatment was again found with these children. At 3- and 6-month follow-up, children receiving the intervention maintained their caloric intake and weight gain.

Children participating in studies by Stark and colleagues consistently increased their daily caloric intake to achieve an average weight gain of 1.47 kg. A meta-analysis comparing the effects of behavioral intervention to medical interventions of parenteral and enteral nutrition found the gains reported for the behavioral treatment to be comparable to medical intervention for weight gain and caloric intake (Jelalian, Stark, Reynolds, & Seifer, 1998).

The fourth study by Stark et al. (2003) compared a nutritional intervention alone to a nutritional plus behavioral intervention. Both interventions consisted of five weekly sessions followed by a final review session. Parents and children were treated separately. Each session focused on a specific meal with information provided on nutrition. Parents were taught child behavior management techniques each week geared toward managing and motivating children to eat the foods presented. Parents were also taught to monitor and reinforce their child's food intake. In the child group, in addition to nutritional information, children practiced weekly calorie goals by eating high-calorie meals in session. Four children received the behavioral intervention, and three received the nutrition education intervention. Data obtained using a multiple-baseline design revealed that the behavioral group had an almost twofold greater increase in daily calorie intake and weight gain by the end of treatment. Calorie intake was maintained at this high level at 2-year follow-up.

Stark and colleagues have conducted a thorough research program designed to increase dietary adherence in children with CF. However, the small number of subjects and the fact that only one investigative team has tested these strategies make behavioral intervention to improve dietary adherence in children with CF only a promising intervention.

Improving Dietary Adherence in Practice

The studies by Stark and colleagues used monitoring and contingency management to increase dietary adherence with information tailored directly to the child. Dr. Stark has made available to purchasers of this book her complete treatment protocol. Detailed procedures for implementing the protocol can be found on the companion Web site to this book. A general overview is provided here.

The first phase of the program is dedicated to careful monitoring and recording of food intake. Stark and colleagues explain to parents that monitoring allows parents to learn the relative calorie intake of many different foods so that eventually parents will be able to effectively identify when their child is meeting his or her calorie goals. Monitoring starts with a 2-week baseline assessment. Parents are provided with necessary measuring devices, including a graduated measuring cup, measuring spoons, and a digital food scale, to ensure accurate recording. Practice in weighing and measuring foods is conducted and followed by teaching parents to calculate calories by using a calorie book and reading food labels. Relatively simple techniques can be used to calculate caloric intake. Alternatively, computer programs exist for these purposes. Detailed monitoring forms are used to record food eaten, how it was prepared, amount served, amount left, amount consumed, and calories.

While parents are being trained in monitoring and recording food intake, their children take part in a separate group. After engaging the children in the group using personalized T-shirts, children are provided with education regarding the importance of nutrition in CF and how the digestive process works. Frequent praise and sticker charts are used to reinforce children's active participation in the group.

Baseline monitoring is used to set each child's individual caloric goals. Then, parents are instructed in how to use behavioral child management skill to encourage eating. This component distinguishes the Stark et al. program from many others in which parents are told what to feed their children, not how to do it. Differential attention to eating, praise for eating, and ignoring noneating behaviors are taught to parents. Sticker charts are also used to reward calorie intake. Rules around eating are implemented (e.g., a 20-minute limit to meal duration), and positive consequences for following mealtime rules and negative consequences for rule violations are reviewed. These rules are also introduced in the children's group. In addition, ways to increase intake are discussed in the group, and contracts regarding intake are established. Eating different foods are also rehearsed in the children's group.

The different components of the protocol are reviewed across multiple sessions to help ensure that the behavior change is consolidated by the parents. This is accomplished by reviewing the procedures to increase intake at breakfast, lunch, dinner, and snack. A detailed problem-solving procedure is used in some sessions in order to help parents learn how to best apply the parenting skills taught for the particular difficulties posed by their child. Other sessions are used to teach parents the best way to introduce new foods to their children and increase calories at mealtimes. The final sessions also review guidelines for diet management on sick days as well as ways to increase caloric consumption following an illness. Children's groups also use a variety of entertaining activities to engage children in the protocol, such as "Energy Bingo," which help children identify high-calorie foods and prepare meals, such as their own pizzas. The last children's group is used to review the program, praise the children for their successes, and have a "graduation" party in which children receive trophies for participation.

Interventions to Improve Adherence to Multiple Components
of the CF Regimen

Several studies have attempted to increase adherence to multiple aspects of the
CF regimen. A psychoeducational program called the Cystic Fibrosis Family
Education Program targeted adherence to self-management across the entire
treatment regimen (Bartholomew et al., 1997). The Cystic Fibrosis Family
Education Program is a self-paced curriculum that provides teaching on all aspects
of self-management in CF and instructs families on the use of goal setting, reinforcement, and self-monitoring. Outcome measures of knowledge, self-efficacy,
and self-management were obtained. Significant effects for self-management
scores were reported, but no objective measures of adherence were obtained.

Goldbeck and Babka (2001) evaluated the impact of a multifamily educational program for children with CF who are 12 years of age or younger. In this
study, 16 families participated in the educational program, both individually and
in multifamily groups, with four to six families in each group. Sessions focused
on a specific management or educational area for CF (e.g., medications, chest
physiotherapy, and nutrition). Members of the medical treatment team participated in these educational sessions. The instructional sessions were alternated
with group discussions and role-plays. No changes were found on any of the
measures of adherence or coping following the educational program, however.

Alexandra Quittner and colleagues have just completed a randomized control study comparing behavioral family systems therapy (BFST) to education
only to improve knowledge about CF, adherence to chest physiotherapy and
medication, and family functioning in adolescents with CF (Quittner, Drotar, &
Ievers-Landis, 2004; Quittner et al., 2000). This study was unique in that it specifically targeted and measured adherence to three separate components of treatment (enzyme use, inhaled medications, and airway clearance) and employed
multiple measures of adherence on each outcome variable, including self-report,
videotaped discussions, and electronic monitoring (Quittner et al., 2000).

Families of children with CF ($N = 120$, of whom 78 completed the study)
across three sites were randomized to BFST, family learning (psychoeducation),
and standard care. Patients in the BFST arm showed significant improvements
in self-reported frequencies and duration of airway clearance by self-report
(Quittner, Drotar, & Ievers-Landis, 2004). Significant differences in knowledge
were seen in the psychoeducation arm of the study. Finally, as expected, the
BFST arm showed significant improvements relative to the other conditions
in family conflict, communication, and problem solving (Quittner, Drotar, &

Ievers-Landis, 2004). The findings from this randomized clinical trial at three sites indicate that BFST is a promising intervention for adherence in CF.

Improving Adherence to Chest Physiotherapy
and Medication in Practice

Quittner et al. (2000) have made their entire treatment manual available for use by readers. Their family-based treatment approach for increasing adolescent adherence to chest physiotherapy and medication is summarized and reviewed here.

BFST is an interactive 11-session protocol focusing on problem solving and communication. The initial session is used to assess family problems related to the CF treatment regimen, as well as other interactional problems in the family, and to develop a general treatment plan. After each session, the teen is given homework assignments (e.g., monitoring treatment areas after the initial session) and rewarded each week for completing homework. Homework is reviewed at the start of each session.

In the second session, the focus is on presenting different styles of parenting with high levels of affection and support combined with moderate control presented as the optimal parenting style. Negotiable and nonnegotiable issues are defined in each family in order to allow the adolescent some opportunity to develop autonomous functioning. Two sessions are used to teach and practice a family problem-solving technique. The technique starts with defining the problem, followed by asking each family member to generate as many solutions as possible. Each family member independently evaluates each solution until the family comes to agreement on a few potential solutions acceptable to all of them. One solution is eventually selected, and then a plan is developed to apply the selected solution.

Positive family communication strategies are the focus of two sessions. Communication skills are practiced in session using a game format in which family members ask each other questions. A handout listing communication skills is used to assist each family member in selecting skills they would like to practice. One session is used to facilitate a family discussion about disclosure of CF-related issues in different social settings.

The final sessions of the protocol are used to assist the family in planning for the future management of CF-related problems and providing a review of the plans that have been implemented by the family to improve treatment adherence. For this latter task, a game format is used in which a family member is asked a question about the progress observed, and the other family members write down what they think the person's answer will be. A booster session is also built into the protocol to review the teen's health, adherence to the CF regimen, and the family's success at solving problems related to treatment. Regular meetings at home among the family members to review how treatments are managed are encouraged as the most effective means of maintaining progress obtained in the BFST protocol.

Research Issues

The demanding nature of the CF regimen suggests that behavior change can result in improved outcomes. However, the empirical literature supporting the efficacy of behavioral intervention is small. In order for CF behavioral intervention research to move from an emerging area to an established area, more studies will need to be conducted. This may prove to be more difficult to accomplish than in other areas of pediatric psychology for several reasons. First, new research groups will need to conduct at least a portion of these new studies to ensure that these intensive interventions can successfully generalize across patients and interventionists. Second, research in this area requires large samples in order to explicate the disease and motivational variables that may moderate intervention outcomes. In addition, the relatively low incidence of CF almost invariably requires multisite studies. Thus, it may be difficult to involve new research groups working independently.

Treatment Manuals

As noted above, Stark and colleagues (Stark, Bowen, et al., 1990; Stark et al., 1993, 1996) have developed and tested a group treatment approach to increase calorie consumption in young children with CF. Quittner, Drotar, Ievers-Landis, and Hoffman (2004) have recently tested a new program to improve adherence to chest physiotherapy and medication in adolescents with CF. Both of these research programs show promise as effective interventions, but neither has been tested by independent investigators. We chose to include these manuals on the book's companion Web site (www.oup.com/us/pediatricpsych) to encourage other clinical researchers to examine the components of these treatment protocols and to consider continuing research with this population. Drs. Stark and Quittner have agreed to make their treatment manuals available so that clinicians can use their protocols in practice and to encourage readers interested in conducting future research in this area to contact them.

References

Adams, C., Dreyer, M., Dinakar, C., & Portnoy, J. (2004). Pediatric asthma: A look at adherence from the patient and family perspective. *Current Asthma and Allergy Reports, 4,* 425–432.

Adams, C., Joseph, K., MacLaren, J., DeMore, M., Koven, L., Detwiler, M., et al. (2004, April). *Parent-youth teamwork in pediatric asthma management.* Poster presented at the National Conference on Child Health Psychology, Charleston, SC.

Adams, L. A., & Rickert, V. I. (1989). Reducing bedtime tantrums: Comparison between positive routines and graduated extinction. *Pediatrics, 84,* 756–759.

Addis, M., Hatgis, C., Soysa, C., & Zaslavsky, I. (1999). The dialectics of manual-based treatment. *Behavior Therapist, 22*(Summer), 130–132.

Addis, M., Wade, W., & Hatgis, C. (1999). Barriers to dissemination of evidence-based practices: Addressing practitioners' concerns about manual-based psychotherapy. *Clinical Psychology: Science and Practice, 6,* 430–441.

Alderfer, M., Labay, L., & Kazak, A. (2003). Brief report: Does posttraumatic stress apply to siblings of childhood cancer survivors? *Journal of Pediatric Psychology, 28,* 281–286.

Allen, K., Elliott, A., & Arndorfer, R. (2002). Behavioral pain management for pediatric headache in primary care. *Children's Health Care, 31,* 175–189.

Allen, K., & Mathews, J. (1998). Behavioral management of recurrent pain in children. In T. S. Watson & F. Gresham (Eds.), *Handbook of child behavior therapy* (pp. 263–285). New York: Plenum Press.

American Psychiatric Association. (1994). *Diagnostic and statistical manual of mental disorders* (4th ed.). Washington, DC: Author.

Anbar, R. (2001). Self-hypnosis for the treatment of functional abdominal pain in childhood. *Clinical Pediatrics, 40,* 447–451.

Anderson, B., Brackett, J., Ho, J., & Laffel, L. (2000). An intervention to promote family teamwork in diabetes management tasks: Relationships among parental involvement, adherence to blood glucose monitoring, and glycemic control in young adolescents with type 1 diabetes. In D. Drotar (Ed.), *Promoting adherence to medical treatment and chronic childhood illness: Concepts, methods, and interventions* (pp. 71–93). Mahwah, NJ: Erlbaum.

Andrasik, F., Grazzi, L., Usai, S., D'Amico, D., Leone, M., & Bussone, G. (2003). Brief neurologist-administered behavioral treatment of pediatric episodic tension-type headache. *Neurology, 60*, 1215–1216.

Arndorfer, R., & Allen, K. (2001). Extending the efficacy of a thermal biofeedback treatment package to the management of tension-type headaches in children. *Headache, 41*, 183–192.

Azrin, N. H., & Besalel, V. A. (1979). *A parent's guide to bedwetting control.* New York: Simon & Schuster.

Azrin, N. H., Sneed, T. J., & Foxx, R. M. (1974). Dry-bed training: Rapid elimination of childhood enuresis. *Behaviour Research and Therapy, 12*, 147–156.

Banez, J., & Cunningham, C. (2003). Pediatric gastrointestinal disorders: Recurrent abdominal pain, inflammatory bowel disease, and rumination disorder/cyclic vomiting. In M. Roberts (Ed.), *Handbook of pediatric psychology* (3rd ed., pp. 462–478). New York: Guilford Press.

Barakat, L., Hetzke, J., Foley, B., Carey, M., Gyato, K., & Phillips, P. (2003). Evaluation of a social skills training group intervention with children treated for brain tumors: A pilot study. *Journal of Pediatric Psychology, 28*, 299–307.

Barrera, M., Chung, J., Greenberg, M., & Fleming, C. (2002). Preliminary investigation of a group intervention for siblings of pediatric cancer patients. *Children's Health Care, 31*, 131–142.

Bartholomew, L. K., Czyewski, D. I., Parcel, G. S., Swank, P. R., Sockrider, M. M., Mariotto, M. J., et al. (1997). Self-management of cystic fibrosis: Short term outcomes of the Cystic Fibrosis Family Education Program. *Health Education and Behavior, 24*, 652–666.

Beidel, D. C., & Turner, S. M. (1998). *Shy children, phobic adults.* Washington, DC: American Psychological Association.

Berkowitz, R., Wadden, T., Tershakovec, A., & Cronquist, J. (2003). Behavior therapy and sibutramine for the treatment of adolescent obesity. *Journal of the American Medical Association, 289*, 1805–1812.

Bernard-Bonnin, A., Haley, N., Belanger, S., & Nadeau, D. (1993). Parent/caregiver and patient perceptions about encopresis and its treatment. *Journal of Developmental and Behavioral Pediatrics, 14*, 397–400.

Bleil, M., Ramesh, S., Miller, B., & Wood, B. (2000). The influence of parent-child relatedness on depressive symptoms in children with asthma: Tests of moderator and mediator models. *Journal of Pediatric Psychology, 25*, 481–491.

Bollard, J., & Nettlebeck, T. (1981). A comparison of Dry Bed Training and standard urine alarm conditioning treatment of childhood bedwetting. *Behaviour Research and Therapy, 19*, 215–226.

Bonner, S., Zimmerman, B., Evans, D., Irigoyen, M., Resnick, D., & Mellins, R. (2002). An individualized intervention to improve asthma management among urban Latino and African-American families. *Journal of Asthma, 39,* 167–179.

Borowitz, S. M., Cox, D. J., Sutphen, J. L., & Kovatchev, B. (2002). Treatment of childhood encopresis: A randomized trial comparing three treatment protocols. *Journal of Pediatric Gastroenterology and Nutrition, 34,* 378–384.

Bradbury, M., & Meadow, S. (1995). Combined treatment with enuresis alarm and desmopressin for nocturnal enuresis. *Acta Paediatrica Scandinavica, 84,* 1014–1018.

Bronfenbrenner, U. (1979). *The ecology of human development.* Cambridge, MA: Harvard University Press.

Brown, K., & Piazza, C. (1999). Commentary: Enhancing the effectiveness of sleep treatments: Develop a functional approach. *Journal of Pediatric Psychology, 29,* 487–489.

Brown, R. (2003). Editorial: The *Journal of Pediatric Psychology* will support the publication of clinical trials. *Journal of Pediatric Psychology, 28,* 173.

Brown, R., Madan-Swain, A., & Lambert, R. (2003). Posttraumatic stress symptoms in adolescent survivors of childhood cancer and their mothers. *Journal of Traumatic Stress, 16,* 309–318.

Butler, R. J., Redfern, E. J., & Forsythe, W. I. (1990). The child's construing of nocturnal enuresis: A method of inquiry and prediction of outcome. *Journal of Child Psychology and Psychiatry, 31,* 447–454.

Cady, R., Farmer, K., Griesemer, K., & Sable, J. (1996). Prevalence of headache in children. *Headache Quarterly, Current Treatment and Research, 7,* 312–318.

Campbell, T., & Patterson, J. (1995). The effectiveness of family interventions in the treatment of physical illness. *Journal of Marital and Family Therapy, 21,* 545–583.

Cassidy, K., Reid, G., McGrath, P., Finley, G., Smith, D., Morley, C., et al. (2002). Watch needle, watch TV: Audiovisual distraction in preschool immunization. *Pain Medicine, 3,* 108–118.

Castonguay, L., Goldfried, M., Wiser, S., Rave, P., & Hayes, A. (1996). Predicting the effect of cognitive therapy for depression: A study of unique and common factors. *Journal of Consulting and Clinical Psychology, 64,* 497–504.

Chadez, L. H., & Nurius, P. S. (1987). Stopping bedtime crying: Treating the child and the parents/caregivers. *Journal of Clinical Child Psychology, 16,* 212–217.

Chambless, D. (1996). In defense of dissemination of empirically supported psychological interventions. *Clinical Psychology: Science and Practice, 3,* 230–235.

Chen, E., Cole, S., & Kato, P. (2004). A review of empirically supported psychosocial interventions for pain and adherence outcomes in sickle cell disease. *Journal of Pediatric Psychology, 29,* 197–204.

Chen, E., Craske, M., Katz, E., Schwartz, E., & Zeltzer, L. (2000). Pain-sensitive temperament: Does it predict procedural distress and response to psychological treatment among children with cancer? *Journal of Pediatric Psychology, 25,* 269–278.

Chen, E., Joseph, M., & Zeltzer, L. (2000). Behavioral and cognitive interventions in the treatment of pain in children. *Pediatric Clinics of North America, 47,* 513–525.

Clarke, G., Lewinsohn, P., & Hops, H. (1990). *Instructor's manual for the adolescent coping with depression course.* Portland, OR: Kaiser Permanente Center for Health Research.

Clay, D., Mordhorst, M., & Lehn, L. (2002). Empirically supported treatments in pediatric psychology: Where is the diversity? *Journal of Pediatric Psychology, 27,* 325–338.

Cohen, L. (2004a). *Coping skills training for school age children.* Unpublished protocol.

Cohen, L. (2004b). *Guidelines for using distraction with preschoolers.* Unpublished protocol.

Cohen, L., Blount, R., Cohen, R., Ball, C., McCleelan, C., & Bernard, R. (2001). Children's expectations and memories of acute distress: Short and long-term efficacy of pain management interventions. *Journal of Pediatric Psychology, 26,* 367–374.

Cox, D. J., Sutphen, J., Borowitz, S., Kovatchev, B., & Ling, W. (1998). Contribution of behavior therapy and biofeedback to laxative therapy in the treatment of pediatric encopresis. *Annals of Behavioral Medicine, 20,* 70–76.

Cox, D. J., Sutphen, J., Ling, W., Quillian, W., & Borowitz, S. (1996). Additive benefits of laxative, toilet training, and biofeedback therapies in the treatment of pediatric encopresis. *Journal of Pediatric Psychology, 21,* 659–670.

Creer, T. (2000). Self-management and the control of chronic pediatric illness. In D. Drotar (Ed.), *Promoting adherence to medical treatment and chronic childhood illness: Concepts, methods, and interventions* (pp. 95–129). Mahwah, NJ: Erlbaum.

Curtis, N., Ronan, K., & Borduin, C. (2004). Multisystemic treatment: A meta-analysis of outcome studies. *Journal of Family Psychology, 18,* 411–419.

Cystic Fibrosis Foundation. (2003, September). *Patient registry 2000 annual data report.* Bethesda, MD: Author.

Dahl, J., Lindquist, B., Tysk, C., Leissner, P., Philipson, L., & Jarnerot, G. (1991). Behavioral medicine treatment in chronic constipation with paradoxical anal sphincter contraction. *Diseases of the Colon and Rectum, 34,* 769–776.

Dahlquist, L., Busby, S., Slifer, K., Tucker, C., Eischen, S., Hilley, L., et al. (2002). Distraction for children of different ages who undergo repeated needlesticks. *Journal of Pediatric Oncology Nursing, 19,* 22–34.

Dahlquist, L., Pendley, J., Landthrip, D., Jones, C., & Steuber, C. (2002). Distraction intervention for preschoolers undergoing intramuscular injections and subcutaneous port access. *Health Psychology, 21,* 94–99.

Dahlquist, L., & Switkin, M. (2003). Chronic and recurrent pain. In M. Roberts (Ed.), *Handbook of pediatric psychology* (3rd ed., pp, 198–215). New York: Guilford Press.

Davis, C., Delamater, A., Shaw, K., La Greca, A., Eidson, M., Perez-Rodriguez, J., et al. (2001). Brief report: Parenting styles, regimen adherence and glycemic control in 4–10 year old children with diabetes. *Journal of Pediatric Psychology, 26,* 123–129.

Deaton, A. (1985). Adaptive noncompliance in pediatric asthma: The parent as expert. *Journal of Pediatric Psychology, 10,* 1–14.

DeCivita, M., & Dobkin, P. (2004). Pediatric adherence as a multidimensional and dynamic construct, involving a triadic partnership. *Journal of Pediatric Psychology, 29,* 157–169.

deJong, P. T., Grevink, R. G., Roorda, R. J., Kaptein, A. A., & van der Schans, G. P. (1994). Effect of a home exercise training program in patients with cystic fibrosis. *Chest, 105,* 463–468.

DeLambo, K., Ievers-Landis, C., Drotar, D., & Quittner, A. (2004). Association of observed family relationship quality and problem-solving skills with treatment adherence in older children and adolescents with cystic fibrosis. *Journal of Pediatric Psychology, 29,* 343–353.

Dolgin, M., Somer, E., Zaidel, N., & Zaizov, R. (1997). A structured group intervention for siblings of children with cancer. *Journal of Child and Adolescent Group Therapy, 7,* 3–18.

Donaldson, D., Spirito, A., & Overholser, J. (2003). Treatment of adolescent suicide attempters. In A. Spirito & J. Overholser (Eds.), *Evaluating and treating adolescent suicide attempters: From research to practice* (pp. 295–321). New York: Academic Press.

Drotar, D. (2002) Enhancing reviews of psychological treatments with pediatric populations: Thoughts on next steps. *Journal of Pediatric Psychology, 27,* 167–176.

Durand, V. M., & Mindell, J. A. (1990). Behavioral treatment of multiple childhood sleep disorders: Effects on child and family. *Behavior Modification, 14,* 37–49.

Eifert, G., Evans, I., & McKendrick, V. (1990). Matching treatments to client problems not diagnostic labels: A case for paradigmatic behavior therapy. *Journal of Behavior Therapy and Experimental Psychology, 21,* 163–172.

Eifert, G., Schulte, D., Zvolensky, M., Lejuez, C., & Lau, A. (1997). Manualized behavior therapy: Merits and challenges. *Behavior Therapy, 28,* 499–509.

El-Anany, F. G., Maghraby, H. A., Shaker, S. E., & Abdel-Moneim, A. M. (1999). Primary nocturnal enuresis: A new approach to conditioning treatment. *Urology, 53,* 405–409.

Ellis, D., Naar-King, S., Frey, M., Rowland, M., & Greger, N. (2003). Case study: Feasibility of multisystemic therapy as a treatment for urban adolescents with poorly controlled Type 1 diabetes. *Journal of Pediatric Psychology, 28,* 287–293.

Engel, G. (1977). The need for a new medical model: A challenge for biomedicine. *Science, 196,* 129–136.

Epstein, L., Paluch, R., Gordy, C., Saelens, B., & Ernst, M. (2000). Problem solving in the treatment of childhood obesity. *Journal of Consulting and Clinical Psychology, 68,* 405–418.

Fanurik, D., Koh, J., & Schmidt, M. (2000). Distraction techniques combined with MELA: Effects on IV insertion pain and distress in children. *Children's Health Care, 29,* 87–101.

Feindler, E., & Ecton, R. (1986). *Adolescent anger control: Cognitive-behavioral techniques.* New York: Pergamon Press.

Ferber, R. (1985). *How to solve your child's sleep problems.* New York: Simon & Schuster.

Fiese, B., & Wamboldt, F. (2000). Family routines, rituals and asthma management: A proposal for family-based strategies to increase treatment adherence. *Families, Systems, and Health, 18,* 405–418.

Fiese, B., Wamboldt, F., & Anbar, R. (2005). Family asthma management rituals: Connections to medical adherence and quality of life. *Journal of Pediatrics, 146,* 171–176.

Finney, J., Lemanek, K., Cataldo, M., Katz, H., & Fuqua, R. W. (1989). Pediatric psychology in primary health care: Brief targeted therapy for recurrent abdominal pain. *Behavior Therapy, 20,* 283–291.

France, K. G. (1992). Behavior characteristics and security in sleep-disturbed infants treated with extinction. *Journal of Pediatric Psychology, 17,* 467–475.

France, K. G., Blampied, N. M., & Wilkinson, P. (1991). Treatment of infant sleep disturbance by trimeprazine in combination with extinction. *Journal of Developmental and Behavioral Pediatrics, 12,* 308–314.

France, K. G., & Hudson, S. M. (1990). Behavior management of infant sleep disturbance. *Journal of Applied Behavioral Analysis, 23,* 91–98.

Friedberg, R., Crosby, L., Friedberg, B., Rutter, J., & Knight, K. R. (2000). Making cognitive-behavioral therapy user-friendly to children. *Cognitive and Behavioral Practice, 6,* 189–200.

Gil, K., Anthony, K., Carson, J., Redding-Lallinger, R., Daeschner, C., & Ware, R. (2001). Daily coping practice predicts treatment effects in children with sickle cell disease. *Journal of Pediatric Psychology, 26,* 163–173.

Gil, K., Carson, J., Sedway, J. W., Porter, L., Schaeffer, J., & Orringer, E. (2000). Follow-up of coping skills training in adults with sickle cell disease: Analysis of daily pain and coping practice diaries. *Health Psychology, 19,* 85–90.

Gil, K. M., Wilson, J. J., Edens, J. L., Webster, D., Abrams, M., Orringer, E., et al. (1996). Effects of cognitive coping skills training on coping strategies and experimental pain sensitivity in African American adults with sickle cell disease. *Health Psychology, 15,* 3–10.

Gil, K. M., Wilson, J. J., Edens, J. L., Workman, E., Ready, J., Sedway, J., et al. (1997). Cognitive coping skills training in children with sickle cell disease pain. *International Journal of Behavioral Medicine, 4,* 364–377.

Godley, S., White, W., Diamond, G., Passetti, L., & Titus, J. (2001). Therapist reactions to manual-guided therapies for the treatment of adolescent marijuana users. *Clinical Psychology: Science and Practice, 8,* 405–417.

Goldbeck, L., & Babka, C. (2001). Development and evaluation of a multi-family psychoeducational program for cystic fibrosis. *Patient Education and Counseling, 44,* 187–192.

Gonzalez, S., Steinglass, P., & Reiss, D. (1989). Putting the illness in its place: Discussion groups for families with chronic medical illness. *Family Process, 28,* 68–87.

Grace, N., Spirito, A., Finch, A. J., & Ott, E. (1993). Coping skills for anxiety control in children. In A. J. Finch, W. M. Nelson, & E. Ott (Eds.), *Cognitive-behavioral procedures with children and adolescents: A practical guide* (pp. 257–288). Boston: Allyn & Bacon.

Greco, P., Pendley, J., McDonell, K., & Reeves, G. (2001). A peer group intervention for adolescents with type 1 diabetes and their best friends. *Journal of Pediatric Psychology, 26,* 485–490.

Hagopian, L. P., & Thompson, R. H. (1999). Reinforcement of compliance with respiratory treatment in a child with cystic fibrosis. *Journal of Applied Behavior Analysis, 32,* 233–236.

Haynes, R. (1979). Introduction. In R. Haynes, D. Taylor, & D. Sackett (Eds.), *Compliance in health care* (p. 1). Baltimore: Johns Hopkins University Press.

Haynes, S., Kaholokula, J. K., & Nelson, K. (1999). The idiographic application of nomothetic empirically based treatments. *Clinical Psychology: Science and Practice, 6,* 456–461.

Henggeler, S. (2003). Commentary on Ellis et al.: Adapting multisystemic therapy for challenging clinical problems of children and adolescents. *Journal of Pediatric Psychology, 28,* 295–297.

Henggeler, S., Schoenwald, S., & Rowland, M. (2002). *Serious emotional disturbance in children and adolescents: Multisystemic therapy.* New York: Guilford Press.

Henin, A., Otto, M., & Reilly-Harrington, N. (2001). Introducing flexibility in manualized treatments: Application of recommended strategies to the cognitive behavioral treatment of bipolar disorder. *Cognitive and Behavioral Practice, 8,* 317–328.

Hiscock, H., & Wake, M. (2002). Randomized controlled trial of behavioral infant sleep intervention to improve infant sleep and maternal mood. *British Medical Journal, 324,* 1062–1067.

Hoekstra-Weebers, J., Heuval, F., Jaspers, J., Kamps, W., & Klip, E. (1998). Brief report: An intervention program for parents of pediatric cancer patients: A randomized controlled trial. *Journal of Pediatric Psychology, 23,* 207–205.

Hoekx, L., Wyndaele, J. J., & Vermandel, A. (1998). The role of bladder biofeedback in the treatment of children with refractory nocturnal enuresis associated with idiopathic detrusor instability and small bladder capacity. *Journal of Urology, 160,* 858–860.

Holden, W., Deichmann, M., & Levy, J. (1999). Empirically supported treatments in pediatric psychology: Recurrent pediatric headache. *Journal of Pediatric Psychology, 24,* 91–109.

Holroyd, R., Penzien, D., Hursey, K., Tobin, D., Rogers, L., Holm, J., et al. (1984). Change mechanisms in EMG biofeedback training: Cognitive changes underlying improvements in tension headache. *Journal of Consulting and Clinical Psychology, 52,* 1039–1053.

Holzer, F. J., Schnall, R., & Laudau, L. I. (1984). The effect of a home exercise programme in children with cystic fibrosis and asthma. *Australian Paediatric Journal, 20,* 297–302.

Houts, A. C., & Abramson, H. (1990). Assessment and treatment for functional childhood enuresis and encopresis: Toward a partnership between health psychologists and physicians. In S. B. Morgan & T. M. Okwumabua (Eds.), *Child and adolescent disorders: Developmental and health psychology perspectives* (pp. 47–103). Hillsdale, NJ: Erlbaum.

Houts, A. C., & Liebert, R. M. (1984). *Bedwetting: A guide for parents and children.* Springfield, IL: Charles C. Thomas.

Houtzager, B. A., Grootenhuis, M. A., & Last, B. F. (2001). Supportive groups for sibs of pediatric oncology patients: Impact on anxiety. *Psycho-Oncology, 10,* 315–324.

Humphreys, P., & Gevirtz, R. (2000). Treatment of recurrent abdominal pain: Components analysis of four treatment protocols. *Journal of Pediatric Gastroenterology and Nutrition, 31,* 47–51.

Jacobson, A., Hauser, S., Lavori, P., Willett, J., Cole, C., Wolfsdorf, J., et al. (1994). Family environment and glycemic control: A four year prospective study of children and adolescents with insulin-dependent diabetes mellitus. *Psychosomatic Medicine, 56,* 401–409.

Janicke, D., & Finney, J. (1999). Empirically supported treatments in pediatric psychology: Recurrent abdominal pain. *Journal of Pediatric Psychology, 24*(2), 115–128.

Jarvelin, M. R. (2000). Commentary: Empirically supported treatments in pediatric psychology: Nocturnal enuresis. *Journal of Pediatric Psychology, 25,* 215–218.

Jarvelin, M. R., Vikevainen-Tervonen, L., Moilanen, I., & Huttunen, N. P. (1988). Enuresis in seven-year-old children. *Acta Paediatrica Scandinavica, 77,* 148–153.

Jelalian, E., & Mehlenbeck, R. (2002). Peer-enhanced weight management treatment for overweight adolescents: Some preliminary findings. *Journal of Clinical Psychology in Medical Settings, 9,* 15–23.

Jelalian, E., & Saelens, B. (1999). Empirically supported treatments in pediatric psychology: Pediatric obesity. *Journal of Pediatric Psychology, 24*(3), 223–248.

Jelalian, E., Stark, L. J., Reynolds, L., & Seifer, R. (1998). Nutrition intervention for weight gain in cystic fibrosis: A meta analysis. *Journal of Pediatrics, 132,* 486–492.

Johnson, C. M., Bradley-Johnson, S., & Stack, J. M. (1981). Decreasing the frequency of infants' nocturnal crying with the use of scheduled awakenings. *Family Practice Research Journal, 1,* 98–104.

Johnson, C. M., & Lerner, M. (1985). Amelioration of infant sleep disturbances: II. Effects of scheduled awakenings by compliant parents/caregivers. *Infant Mental Health Journal, 6,* 21–30.

Kainz, K. (2002). A behavioral conditioning program for treatment of nocturnal enuresis. *Behavior Therapist, 25,* 185–187.

Kamps, J., Rapoff, M., & Roberts, M. (2004, April). *Exploring outcomes of an asthma adherence intervention.* Poster presented at the National Conference on Child Health Psychology, Charleston, SC.

Kashikar-Zuck, S., Swain, N. F., Jones, B. A., & Graham, T. B. (in press). Efficacy of cognitive-behavioral intervention in juvenile primary fibromyalgia syndrome. *Journal of Rheumatology.*

Kaslow, N., & Brown, F. (1995). Culturally sensitive family interventions for chronically ill youth: Sickle cell disease as an example. *Family Systems Medicine, 13,* 201–213.

Kaslow, N., Collins, M., Loundy, M., Brown, F., Hollins, L., & Eckman, J. (1997). Empirically validated family interventions for pediatric psychology: Sickle cell disease as an exemplar. *Journal of Pediatric Psychology, 22,* 213–227.

Kaslow, N., Collins, M., Rashid, F., Baskin, M., Griffith, J., Hollins, L., et al. (2000). The efficacy of a pilot family psychoeducational intervention for pediatric sickle cell disease. *Families, Systems and Health, 18,* 381–404.

Kataria, S., Swanson, M. S., & Trevathan, G. E. (1987). Persistence of sleep disturbances in preschool children. *Behavioral Pediatrics, 110,* 642–646.

Kazak, A. (1989). Families of chronically ill children: A systems and social ecological model of adaptation and challenge. *Journal of Consulting and Clinical Psychology, 57,* 25–30.

Kazak, A. (2002a). Challenges in family health intervention research. *Families, Systems and Health, 20,* 51–59.

Kazak, A. (2002b). *Journal of Pediatric Psychology* (JPP)—1998–2002: Editor's vale dictum. *Journal of Pediatric Psychology, 27,* 653–663.

Kazak, A. (2003a). Family assessment. In T. Ollendick & C. Schroeder (Eds.), *Encyclopedia of pediatric and child clinical psychology* (pp. 231–232). New York: Kluwer Academic/Plenum.

Kazak, A. (2003b). Family intervention. In T. Ollendick & C. Schroeder (Eds.), *Encyclopedia of pediatric and child clinical psychology* (p. 233). New York: Kluwer Academic/Plenum.

Kazak, A. (2005). Evidence-based interventions for survivors of childhood cancer and their families. *Journal of Pediatric Psychology, 30,* 29–39.

Kazak, A., Alderfer, M., Rourke, M., Simms, S., Streisand, R., & Grossman, J. (2004). Posttraumatic stress symptoms (PTSS) and posttraumatic stress disorder (PTSD) in families of adolescent childhood cancer survivors. *Journal of Pediatric Psychology, 29,* 211–219.

Kazak, A., Alderfer, M., Streisand, R., Simms, S., Rourke, M., Barakat, L., et al. (2004). Treatment of posttraumatic stress symptoms in adolescent survivors of childhood cancer and their families: A randomized clinical trial. *Journal of Family Psychology, 18,* 493–504.

Kazak, A., Barakat, L., Alderfer, M., Rourke, M., Meeske, K., Gallagher, P., et al. (2001). Posttraumatic stress in survivors of childhood cancer and mothers: Development and validation of the Impact of Traumatic Stressors Interview Schedule (ITSIS). *Journal of Clinical Psychology in Medical Settings, 8,* 307–323.

Kazak, A., Barakat, L., Meeske, K., Christakis, D., Meadows, A., Casey, R., et al. (1997). Posttraumatic stress, family functioning, and social support in survivors of childhood leukemia and their mothers and fathers. *Journal of Consulting and Clinical Psychology, 65,* 120–129.

Kazak, A., Blackall, G., Boyer, B., Brophy, P., Buzaglo, J., Penati, B., et al. (1996). Implementing a pediatric leukemia intervention for procedural pain: The impact on staff. *Families, Systems and Health, 14,* 43–56.

Kazak, A., Blackall, G., Himelstein, B., Brophy, P., & Daller, R. (1995). Producing systemic change in pediatric practice: An intervention protocol for reducing distress during painful procedures. *Family Systems Medicine, 13,* 173–185.

Kazak, A., & Kunin-Batson, A. (2001). Psychological and integrative interventions in pediatric procedural pain. In G. A. Findley & P. McGrath (Eds.), *Acute and procedural pain in infants and children* (pp. 77–100). Seattle, WA: ISAP Press.

Kazak, A., Penati, B., Brophy, P., & Himelstein, B. (1998). Pharmacologic and psychologic interventions for procedural pain. *Pediatrics, 102,* 59–66.

Kazak, A., Rourke, M., & Crump, T. (2003). Families and other systems in pediatric psychology. In M. Roberts (Ed.), *Handbook of pediatric psychology* (3rd ed., pp. 159–175). New York: Guilford Press.

Kazak, A., Simms, S., Alderfer, M., Rourke, M., Crump, T., McClure, K., et al. (in press). Feasibility and preliminary outcomes from a pilot study of a brief psychological intervention for families of children newly diagnosed with cancer. *Journal of Pediatric Psychology.*

Kazak, A., Simms, S., Barakat, L., Hobbie, W., Foley, B., Golomb, B., & Best, M. (1999). Surviving Cancer Competently Intervention Program (SCCIP): A cognitive-behavioral and family therapy intervention for adolescent survivors of childhood cancer and their families. *Family Process, 38,* 175–192.

Kazak, A., Simms, S., & Rourke, M. (2002). Family systems practice in pediatric psychology. *Journal of Pediatric Psychology, 27,* 133–143.

Kazdin, A. E., Kratochwill, T., & VandenBos, G. (1986). Beyond clinical trials: Generalizing from research to practice. *Professional Psychology: Research and Practice, 17,* 391–398.

Keating, J., Butz, R., Burke, E., & Heimberg, R. (1983). Dry-bed training without a urine alarm: Lack of effect of setting and therapist contact with child. *Journal of Behaviour Therapy and Experimental Psychiatry, 14,* 109–115.

Kendall, P. (1998). Directing misperceptions: Researching the issues facing manual-based treatments. *Clinical Psychology: Science and Practice, 5,* 396–399.

Kendall, P., & Chu, B. (2000). Retrospective self-reports of therapist flexibility in a manual-based treatment for youths with anxiety disorders. *Journal of Consulting and Clinical Psychology, 29,* 209–220.

Kendall, P., Chu, B., Gifford, A., Hayes, C., & Nauta, M. (1998). Breathing life into a manual: Flexibility and creativity with manual-based treatments. *Cognitive and Behavioral Practice, 5,* 177–198.

Kendall, P., Kipnis, D., & Otto-Salaj, L. (1992). When clients don't progress: Influence on and explanation for lack of therapeutic process. *Cognitive Therapy and Research, 16,* 269–282.

Kennard, B., Stewart, S., Olvera, R., Bawdon, R., OhAilin, A., Lewis, C., et al. (2004). Nonadherence in adolescent oncology patients: Preliminary data on psychological risk factors and relationships to outcome. *Journal of Clinical Psychology in Medical Settings, 11,* 31–39.

Kerwin, M. L. (1999). Empirically supported treatments in pediatric psychology: Severe feeding problems. *Journal of Pediatric Psychology, 24*(3), 194–213.

Kleiber, C., Craft-Rosenberg, M., & Harper, D. (2001). Parents as distraction coaches during IV insertion: A randomized study. *Journal of Pain and Symptom Management, 22,* 851–861.

Koeppen, A. S. (1974). Relaxation training for children. *Journal of Elementary School Guidance and Counseling, 9,* 14–21.

Koontz, K., Short, A., Kalinyak, K., & Noll, R. (2004). A randomized, controlled pilot trial of a school intervention for children with sickle cell anemia. *Journal of Pediatric Psychology, 29,* 7–17.

Kroener-Herwig, B., & Denecke, H. (2002). Cognitive-behavioral therapy of pediatric headache: Are there difference in efficacy between a therapist-administered group training and a self-help format? *Journal of Psychosomatic Research, 53,* 1107–1114.

Kuhn, B., & Elliott, A. (2003). Treatment efficacy in behavioral pediatric sleep medicine. *Journal of Psychosomatic Research, 54,* 587–597.

Kuppenheimer, W., & Brown, R. (2002). Painful procedures in pediatric cancer: A comparison of interventions. *Clinical Psychology Review, 22,* 753–786.

Laffel, L., Vangsness, L., Connell, A., Goebel-Fabbri, A., Butler, D., & Anderson, B. (2003). Impact of ambulatory, family focused teamwork intervention on glycemic control in youth with type 1 diabetes. *Journal of Pediatrics, 142,* 409–416.

La Greca, A. (1990). Issues in adherence with pediatric regimens. *Journal of Pediatric Psychology, 15,* 423–436.

La Greca, A. (1997). Reflections and perspectives on pediatric psychology: Editor's vale dictum. *Journal of Pediatric Psychology, 22,* 759–770.

Lawton, C., France, K. G., & Blampied, N. M. (1991). Treatment of infant sleep disturbance by graduated extinction. *Child and Family Behavior Therapy, 13,* 39–56.

Lemanek, K., Kamps, J., & Chung, N. (2001). Empirically support treatments in pediatric psychology: Regimen adherence. *Journal of Pediatric Psychology, 26,* 253–275.

Levine, M. (1975). Children with encopresis: A descriptive analysis. *Pediatrics, 56,* 412–416.

Lobato, D., & Kao, B. (2001). Sibling-parent group intervention to improve sibling knowledge and adjustment to chronic illness and disability. *Journal of Pediatric Psychology, 26,* 435–453.

Loening-Baucke, V. A. (1989). Factors determining outcome in children with chronic constipation and fecal soiling. *Gut, 30,* 999–1006.

Loening-Baucke, V. A. (1990). Modulation of abnormal defecation dynamics by biofeedback treatment in chronically constipated children with encopresis. *Journal of Pediatrics, 116,* 214–222.

Loening-Baucke, V. A. (1993). Chronic constipation in children. *Gastroenterology, 105,* 1557–1564.

Loening-Baucke, V. A. (2002). Encopresis. *Current Opinions in Pediatrics, 14,* 570–575.

Longabaugh, R., & Wirtz, P. (2001). *Project MATCH hypotheses: Results and causal chain analyses.* Bethesda, MD: U.S. Department of Health and Human Services.

MacLaren, J., & Cohen, L. (in press). A comparison of distraction strategies for venipuncture distress in children. *Journal of Pediatric Psychology.*

Manimala, M., Blount, R., & Cohen, L. (2000). The effects of parental reassurance versus distraction on child distress and coping during immunizations. *Children's Health Care, 29,* 161–177.

Manne, S., DuHamel, K., Gallelli, K., Sorgen, K., & Redd, W. (1998). Posttraumatic stress disorder among mothers of pediatric cancer survivors: Diagnosis, comorbidity, and utility of the PTSD checklists as a screening instrument. *Journal of Pediatric Psychology, 23,* 357–366.

Manne, S., DuHamel, K., Nereo, N., Ostroff, J., Parsons, S., Martini, R., et al. (2002). Predictors of PTSD in mothers of children undergoing bone marrow transplantation: The role of cognitive and social processes. *Journal of Pediatric Psychology, 27,* 607–617.

Marcus, M., Levine, M., & Kalarchian, M. (2003). Cognitive behavioral interventions in the management of severe pediatric obesity. *Cognitive and Behavioral Practice, 10,* 147–156.

Mason, S., Johnson, M., & Woolley, C. (1999). A comparison of distractors for controlling distress in young children during medical procedures. *Journal of Clinical Psychology in Medical Settings, 6,* 239–248.

McDaniel, S., Hepworth, J., & Doherty, W. (1992). *Medical family therapy.* New York: Basic Books.

McFarlane, W. (2002). *Multifamily groups in the treatment of severe psychiatric disorders.* New York: Guilford Press.

McGrath, M., Mellon, M., & Murphy, L. (2000). Empirically supported treatments in pediatric psychology: Constipation and encopresis. *Journal of Pediatric Psychology, 25,* 225–254.

McGrath, P. J., & Feldman, W. (1986). Clinical approach to recurrent abdominal pain in children. *Developmental and Behavioral Pediatrics, 7,* 56–61.

McGrath, P. J., Humphreys, P., Keene, D., Goodman, J., Lascelles, M., Cunningham, S., et al. (1992). The efficacy and efficiency of a self-administered treatment for adolescent migraine. *Pain, 49,* 321–324.

McQuaid, E., & Nassau, J. (1999). Empirically supported treatments in pediatric psychology: Asthma, diabetes, and cancer. *Journal of Pediatric Psychology, 24*, 305–328.

Meichenbaum, D. (1976). Toward a cognitive theory of self-control. In G. Schwartz & D. Shapiro (Eds.), *Consciousness and self-regulation: Advances in research* (pp. 223–260). New York: Plenum Press.

Mellon, M. W., & Houts, A. C. (1998). Home based treatment for primary enuresis. In J. Briesmeister & C. E. Schaefer (Eds.), *Handbook of parent training: Parents as co-therapists for children's behavior problems* (2nd ed., pp. 384–417). New York: Wiley.

Mellon, M. W., & McGrath, M. (2000). Empirically supported treatments in pediatric psychology: Nocturnal enuresis. *Journal of Pediatric Psychology, 25*, 193–214.

Meltzer, L., & Mindell, J. (2004). Nonpharmacologic treatments for pediatric sleeplessness. *Pediatric Clinics of North America, 51*, 1–14.

Micucci, J. (1998). *The adolescent in family therapy: Breaking the cycle of conflict and control.* New York: Guilford Press.

Miller, B., & Wood, B. (1994). Psychophysiologic reactivity in asthmatic children: A cholinergically mediated confluence of pathways. *Journal of American Academy of Child and Adolescent Psychiatry, 33*, 1236–1245.

Minde, K. (1999). Commentary: Empirically supported treatments in pediatric psychology: Bedtime refusal and night wakings in young children. *Journal of Pediatric Psychology, 24*, 483–484.

Mindell, J. (1999). Empirically supported treatments in pediatric psychology: Bedtime refusal and night wakings in young children. *Journal of Pediatric Psychology, 24*, 465–481.

Mindell, J. A., & Durand, V. M. (1993). Treatment of childhood sleep disorders: Generalization across disorders and effects on family members. *Journal of Pediatric Psychology, 18*, 731–750.

Mindell, J. A., Moline, M. L., Zendell, S. M., Brown, L. B., & Fry, J. M. (1994). Pediatricians and sleep disorders: Training and practice. *Pediatrics, 94*, 194–200.

Minuchin, S., Baker, L., Rosman, B., Liebman, R., Millman, L., & Todd, T. (1975). A conceptual model of psychosomatic illness in children: Family organization and family therapy. *Archives of General Psychiatry, 32*, 1031–1038.

Minuchin, S., Rosman, B., & Baker, L. (1978). *Psychosomatic families.* Cambridge, MA: Harvard University Press.

Monti, P. M., Kadden, R., Rohsenow, D. J., Cooney, N., & Abrams, D. (2002). *Treating alcohol dependence: A coping skills training guide* (2nd ed.). New York: Guilford Press.

Nelson-Gray, R., Herbert, D., Sigmon, S., & Brannon, S. (1989). Effectiveness of matched, mismatched, and package treatments of depression. *Journal of Behavior Therapy and Experimental Psychiatry, 20*, 281–294.

Nolan, T., Catto-Smith, T., Coffey, C., & Wells, J. (1998). Randomized controlled trial of biofeedback training in persistent encopresis with anismus. *Archives of Diseases in Childhood, 79*, 131–135.

Nolan, T., Debelle, G., Oberklaid, F., & Coffey, C. (1991). Randomised trial of laxatives in treatment of childhood encopresis. *Lancet, 338*, 523–527.

Ollendick, T. H., & Cerny, J. A. (1981). *Clinical behavior therapy with children.* New York: Plenum Press.

O'Riordan, M. A., Traore, F., Myers, C., Groth, K., Hoff, A., Angiolillo, A., et al. (2004, October). *How low is too low? The use of cluster analysis to define low levels of mercaptopurine metabolites.* Presented at the Third Annual International Conference: Frontiers in Cancer Prevention Research, Seattle, WA.

Ostroff, J., & Steinglass, P. (1996). Psychosocial adaptation following treatment: A family systems perspective on childhood cancer survivorship. In L. Baider, C. Cooper, & A. De-Nour (Eds.), *Cancer and the family* (pp. 127–145). New York: Wiley.

Partin, J., Hamill, S., & Fischel, J. (1992). Painful defecation and fecal soiling in children. *Pediatrics, 89*, 1007–1009.

Pashankar, D., Loening-Baucke, V., & Bishop, W. (2003). Safety of polyethylene glycol 3350 for treatment of chronic constipation in children. *Archives of Pediatric and Adolescent Medicine, 157*, 661–664.

Persons, J. B. (1991). Psychotherapy outcome studies do not accurately represent current models of psychopathology. *American Psychologist, 46*, 99–106.

Persons, J. B., Bostrom, A., & Bertagnolli, A. (1999). Results of randomized controlled trials of cognitive therapy for depression generalize to private practice. *Cognitive Therapy and Research, 23*, 535–548.

Piazza, C., & Fisher, W. (1991). A faded bedtime with response cost protocol for treatment of multiple sleep problems in children. *Journal of Applied Behavioral Analysis, 24*, 129–140.

Piazza, C., Fisher, W., & Sherer, M. (1997). Treatment of multiple sleep problems in children with developmental disabilities: Faded bedtime with response versus bedtime scheduling. *Developmental Medicine and Child Neurology, 39*, 414–418.

Plante, W., Lobato, D., & Engel, R. (2001). Review of group interventions for pediatric chronic conditions. *Journal of Pediatric Psychology, 26*, 435–453.

Pollock, J. I. (1992). Predictors and long-term associations of reported sleep difficulties in infancy. *Journal of Reproductive and Infant Psychology, 10*, 151–168.

Pollock, J. I. (1994). Night waking at five years of age: Predictors and prognosis. *Journal of Child Psychology and Child Psychiatry and Allied Disciplines, 35*, 699–708.

Power, T., DuPaul, G., Shapiro, E., & Kazak, A. (2003). *Promoting children's health: Integrating school, family and community.* New York: Guilford Press.

Powers, S. (1999). Empirically supported treatments in pediatric psychology: Procedure-related pain. *Journal of Pediatric Psychology, 24*, 131–145.

Powers, S., Mitchell, M., Byars, K., Bentti, A., LeCates, S., & Hershey, A. (2001). A pilot study of one-session biofeedback training in pediatric headache. *Neurology, 56,* 133.

Powers, S., Mitchell, M., Graumlich, S., Byars, K., & Kalinyak, K. (2002). Longitudinal assessment of pain, coping, and daily functioning in children with sickle cell disease receiving pain management skills training. *Journal of Clinical Psychology in Medical Settings, 9,* 109–119.

Powers, S., & Spirito, A. (1998). Relaxation training. In N. Alessi, J. T. Coyle, S. Harrison, & S. Eth (Eds.), *Handbook of child and adolescent psychiatry* (Vol. 6, pp. 411–417). New York: John Wiley & Sons.

Pretlow, R. (1999). Treatment of nocturnal enuresis with an ultrasound bladder volume controlled alarm device. *Journal of Urology, 162,* 1224–1228.

Prevatt, F., Heffer, R., & Lowe, P. (2000). A review of school reintegration programs for children with cancer. *Journal of School Psychology, 38,* 447–467.

Pringle, B., Hilley, L., Gelfand, K., Dahlquist, L., Switkin, M., Diver, T., et al. (2001). Decreasing child distress during needle sticks and maintaining treatment gains over time. *Journal of Clinical Psychology in Medical Settings, 8,* 119–130.

Pritchard, A., & Appleton, P. (1988). Management of sleep problems in preschool children. *Early Child Development and Care, 34,* 277–290.

Quittner, A., Drotar, D., Ievers-Landis, C., & Hoffman, S. J. (2004). *Behavioral family systems therapy—(BFST) for teenagers with cystic fibrosis and their parents.* Unpublished manuscript.

Quittner, A. L., Drotar, D., & Ievers-Landis, C. (2004, April). *Improving adherence in adolescents with cystic fibrosis: Comparisons of family therapy and psychoeducation.* Paper presented at the National Conference on Child Health Psychology, Charleston, SC.

Quittner, A. L., Drotar, D., Ievers-Landis, C., Slocum, N., Seidner, D., & Jacobsen, J. (2000). Adherence to medical treatments in adolescents with cystic fibrosis: The development and evaluation of family-based interventions. In D. Drotar (Ed.), *Promoting adherence to medical treatment in chronic childhood illness: Concepts, methods, and interventions* (pp. 383–407). Mahwah, NJ: Erlbaum.

Rapoff, M., Belmont, J., Lindsley, C., Olson, N., Morris, J., & Padur, J. (2002). Prevention of nonadherence to nonsteroidal anti-inflammatory medications for newly diagnosed patients with juvenile rheumatoid arthritis. *Health Psychology, 21,* 620–623.

Rapoff, M. A., Christophersen, E. R., & Rapoff, K. E. (1982). The management of common childhood bedtime problems by pediatric nurse practitioners. *Journal of Pediatric Psychology, 7,* 179–196.

Reid, M. J., Walter, A. L., & O'Leary, S. (1999). Treatment of young children's bedtime refusal and nighttime wakings: A comparison of "standard" and graduated ignoring procedures. *Journal of Abnormal Child Psychology, 27,* 5–16.

Rickert, V. I., & Johnson, C. M. (1988). Reducing nocturnal awakening and crying episodes in infants and young children: A comparison between scheduled awakenings and systematic ignoring. *Pediatrics, 81,* 203–212.

Riekert, K., & Drotar, D. (2000). Adherence to medical treatment in pediatric chronic illness: Critical issues and answered questions. In D. Drotar (Ed.), *Promoting adherence to medical treatment and chronic childhood illness: Concepts, methods, and interventions* (pp. 3–32). Mahwah, NJ: Erlbaum.

Ritterband, L., Cox, D. J., Walker, L., Kovatchev, B., McKnight, L., Patel, V., et al. (2003). An Internet intervention as adjunctive therapy for pediatric encopresis. *Journal of Consulting and Clinical Psychology, 71,* 910–917.

Roberts, M. (1992). Vale dictum: An editor's view of the field of pediatric psychology. *Journal of Pediatric Psychology, 17,* 785–805.

Robin, A. L., & Foster, S. L. (1984). Problem-solving communication training: A behavioral–family systems approach to parent–adolescent conflict. In P. A. Karoly & J. J. Steffen (Eds.), *Adolescent behavior disorders: Foundations and contemporary concerns.* Lexington, MA: D. C. Heath.

Robins, P., Smith, S., Glutting, J., & Bishop, C. (in press). A randomized controlled trial of a cognitive-behavioral intervention for pediatric recurrent abdominal pain. *Journal of Pediatric Psychology.*

Sadeh, A. (1994). Assessment and intervention for infant night waking: Parental reports and activity-based home monitoring. *Journal of Consulting and Clinical Psychology, 62,* 63–68.

Sadeh, A. (1996). Evaluating night wakings in sleep-disturbed infants: A methodological study of parental reports and actigraphy. *Sleep, 19,* 757–762.

Sahler, O. J., Fairclough, D., Phipps, S., Mulhern, R., Dolgin, M., Noll, R., et al. (2005). Using problem-solving skills to reduce negative affectivity in mothers of children with newly diagnosed cancer: Report of a multi-site randomized trial. *Journal of Consulting and Clinical Psychology, 73,* 272–283.

Sahler, O. J., Varni, J., Fairclough, D., Butler, R., Noll, R., Dolgin, M., et al. (2002). Problem-solving skills training for mothers of children with newly diagnosed cancer: A randomized trial. *Journal of Developmental and Behavioral Pediatrics, 23,* 77–86.

Sanders, M., Rebgetz, M., Morrison, M., Bor, W., Gordon, A., Dadds, M., et al. (1989). Cognitive behavioral treatment of recurrent nonspecific abdominal pain in children: An analysis of generalization, maintenance and side effects. *Journal of Consulting and Clinical Psychology, 57,* 294–300.

Sanders, M., Shepherd, R., Cleghorn, G., & Woolford, H. (1994). The treatment of recurrent abdominal pain in children: A controlled comparison of cognitive-behavioral family intervention and standard pediatric care. *Journal of Consulting and Clinical Psychology, 62,* 306–314.

Satin, W., La Greca, A., Zigo, M., & Skyler, J. (1989). Diabetes in adolescence: Effects of multifamily group intervention and parent simulation of diabetes. *Journal of Pediatric Psychology, 14,* 259–569.

Scharff, L., Marcus, D., & Masek, B. (2002). A controlled study of minimal-contact thermal biofeedback treatment in children with migraine. *Journal of Pediatric Psychology, 27,* 109–119.

Schiff, W., Holtz, K., Peterson, N., & Rakusan, T. (2001). Effect of an intervention to reduce procedural pain and distress for children with HIV infection. *Journal of Pediatric Psychology, 26,* 417–427.

Schmitt, B. D. (1987). *Your child's health.* New York: Bantam Books.

Schneiderman-Walker, J., Pollock, S. L., Corey, M., Wilkes, D. D., Canny, G. J., Pedder, L., et al. (2000). A randomized controlled trial of a 3-year home exercise program in cystic fibrosis. *Journal of Pediatrics, 136,* 304–310.

Schulte, D., & Eifert, G. (2002). What to do when manuals fail? The dual model of psychotherapy. *Clinical Psychology: Science and Practice, 9,* 312–328.

Seagull, E. (2000). Beyond mothers and children: Finding the family in pediatric psychology. *Journal of Pediatric Psychology, 25,* 161–169.

Seymour, F. W., Bayfield, G., Brock, P., & During, M. (1983). Management of night-waking in young children. *Australian Journal of Family Therapy, 4,* 217–222.

Seymour, F. W., Brock, P., During, M., & Poole, G. (1989). Reducing sleep disruptions in young children: Evaluation of therapist-guided and written information approaches: A brief report. *Journal of Child Psychology and Psychiatry and Allied Disciplines, 30,* 913–918.

Sharpe, D., & Rossiter, L. (2002). Siblings of children with a chronic illness: A meta-analysis. *Journal of Pediatric Psychology, 27,* 699–710.

Slifer, K., Tucker, C., & Dahlquist, L. (2002). Helping children and caregivers cope with repeated invasive procedures: How are we doing? *Journal of Clinical Psychology in Medical Settings, 9,* 131–152.

Sommers-Flanagan, J., & Sommers-Flanagan, R. (1995). Psychotherapeutic techniques with treatment-resistant adolescents. *Psychotherapy, 32,* 131–140.

Spirito, A. (1999). Introduction: Series on empirically supported treatments in pediatric psychology. *Journal of Pediatric Psychology, 24,* 87–90.

Staiano, A., Andreotti, M. R., Greco, L., Basile, P., & Auricchio, S. (1994). Long-term follow-up of children with chronic idiopathic constipation *Digestive Diseases and Sciences, 39,* 561–564.

Stark, L. (2000). Adherence to diet in chronic conditions. In D. Drotar (Ed.), *Promoting adherence to medical treatment and chronic childhood illness* (pp. 409–427). Mahwah, NJ: Erlbaum.

Stark, L. (2003). Can nutrition counseling be more behavioral? Lessons learned from the dietary management of cystic fibrosis. *Proceedings of the Nutrition Society, 62,* 793–799.

Stark, L. J., Bowen, A. M., Tyc, V. L., Evans, S., & Passero, M. A. (1990). A behavioral approach to increasing calorie consumption in children with cystic fibrosis. *Journal of Pediatric Psychology, 15,* 309–326.

Stark, L. J., Knapp, L. G., Bowen, A. M., Powers, S. W., Jelalian, E., Evans, S., et al. (1993). Increasing calorie consumption in children with cystic fibrosis: Replication with 2-year follow-up. *Journal of Applied Behavior Analysis, 26,* 435–450.

Stark, L. J., Miller, S. T., Plienes, A. J., & Drabman, R. S. (1987). Behavioral contracting to increase chest physiotherapy. *Behavior Modification, 11,* 75–86.

Stark, L. J., Mulvihill, M. M., Powers, S. W., Jelalian, E., Keating, K., Creveling, S., et al. (1996). Behavioral intervention to improve calorie intake of children with cystic fibrosis: Treatment versus wait list control. *Journal of Pediatric Gastroenterology and Nutrition, 22,* 240–253.

Stark, L. J., Opipari, L. C., Donaldson, D. L., Danovsky, M. B., Rasile, D. A., & DelSanto, A. F. (1997). Evaluation of a standard protocol for retentive encopresis: A replication. *Journal of Pediatric Psychology, 22,* 619–633.

Stark, L. J., Opipari, L., Spieth, L., Jelalian, E., Quittner, A., Higgins, L., et al. (2003). Contribution of behavior therapy to dietary treatment in cystic fibrosis: A randomized controlled study with 2-year follow up. *Behavior Therapy, 34,* 237–258.

Stark, L. J., Owens-Stively, J., Spirito, A., Lewis, A., & Guevremont, D. (1990). Group treatment of retentive encopresis. *Journal of Pediatric Psychology, 15,* 659–671.

Starr, P. (1982). *The social transformation of American medicine.* New York: Basic Books.

Stein, H., & Pontious, J. (1985). Family and beyond: The larger context of noncompliance. *Family Systems Medicine, 3,* 179–189.

Steinberg, L., & Levine, A. (1990). *You and your adolescent: A parent's guide for ages 10 to 20* (pp. 156–181). New York: Harper & Row.

Steinglass, P. (1998). Multiple family discussion groups for patients with chronic medical illness. *Families, Systems and Health, 16,* 55–70.

Steinglass, P., Gonzales, S., Dosovitz, I., & Reiss, D. (1982). Discussion groups for chronic hemodialysis patients and their families. *General Hospital Psychiatry, 4,* 7–14.

Streisand, R., Rodrigue, J., Houck, C., Graham-Pole, J., & Berlant, N. (2000). Brief report: Parents of children undergoing bone marrow transplantation: Documenting stress and piloting a psychological intervention program. *Journal of Pediatric Psychology, 25,* 331–337.

Strosahl, K. (1998). The dissemination of manual-based psychotherapies in managed care: Promises, problems and prospects. *Clinical Psychology: Science and Practice, 5,* 382–386.

Sukhai, R. N., Mol, J., & Harris, A. S. (1989). Combined therapy of enuresis alarm and desmopressin in the treatment of nocturnal enuresis. *European Journal of Pediatrics, 148,* 465–467.

Svoren, B., Butler, D., Levine, B., Anderson, B., & Laffel, L. (2003). Reducing acute adverse outcomes in youth with type 1 diabetes mellitus: A randomized controlled trial. *Pediatrics, 112,* 914–922.

Thomas, V., Gruen, R., & Shu, S. (2001). Cognitive behavioral therapy for the management of sickle cell disease pain: Identification and assessment of costs. *Ethnicity and Health, 6,* 59–67.

Thomas, V., Wilson-Barnett, J., & Goodhart, F. (1998). The role of cognitive-behavioral therapy in the management of pain in patients with sickle cell disease. *Journal of Advanced Nursing, 27,* 1002–1009.

Tucker, C., Petersen, S., Herman, K., Fennell, R., Bowling, B., Pedersen, T., et al. (2001). Self regulation predictors of medication adherence among ethnically different pediatric patients with renal transplants. *Journal of Pediatric Psychology, 26,* 455–464.

Varni, J., Katz, E., Colegrove, R., & Dolgin, M. (1993). The impact of social skills training on the adjustment of children with newly diagnosed cancer. *Journal of Pediatric Psychology, 18,* 751–767.

Viswanathan, V., Bridges, S., Whitehouse, W., & Newton, R. (1998). Childhood headaches: Discrete entities or continuum? *Developmental Medicine and Child Neurology, 40,* 544–550.

Walco, G., Sterling, C., Conte, P., & Engel, R. (1999). Empirically supported treatments in pediatric psychology: Disease-related pain. *Journal of Pediatric Psychology, 24*(2), 155–167.

Walco, G., Varni, J., & Ilowite, N. (1992). Cognitive-behavioral pain management in children with juvenile rheumatoid arthritis. *Pediatrics, 89,* 1075–1079.

Wald, A., Chandra, R., Gabel, S., & Chiponis, D. (1987). Evaluation of biofeedback in childhood encopresis. *Journal of Pediatric Gastroenterology and Nutrition, 6,* 554–558.

Walker, J., Johnson, S., Manion, I., & Cloutier, P. (1996). Emotionally focused marital intervention for couples with chronically ill children. *Journal of Consulting and Clinical Psychology, 64,* 1029–1036.

Walker, L. (1999). The evolution of research on recurrent abdominal pain: History, assumptions, and a conceptual model. In P. J. McGrath & G. A. Finley (Eds.), *Progress in pain research and management: Vol. 13. Chronic and recurrent pain in children and adolescents* (pp. 141–172). Seattle, WA. IASP Press.

Wamboldt, M., & Levin, L. (1995). Utility of multifamily psychoeducational groups for medically ill children and adolescents. *Family Systems Medicine, 13,* 151–161.

Weisz, J. (1998). Empirically-supported treatments for children and adolescents. In K. Dobson & K. Craig (Eds.), *Empirically supported therapies: Best practice in professional psychology* (pp. 66–92). Thousand Oaks, CA: Sage.

Weisz, J., Donenberg, G., Han, S., & Weiss, B. (1995). Bridging the gap between laboratory and clinic in child and adolescent psychotherapy. *Journal of Consulting and Clinical Psychology, 63,* 688–701.

Wexler, D. B. (1991). *The PRISM workbook: A program for innovative self-management.* New York: Norton.

Wilson, G. T. (1997). Treatment manuals in clinical practice. *Behavior Research and Therapy, 35,* 205–210.

Wilson, G. T. (1998). Manual-based treatments and clinical practice. *Clinical Psychology: Science and Practice, 5,* 363–375.

Wood, B. (1995). A developmental biopsychosocial approach to the treatment of chronic illness in children and adolescents. In R. H. Mikesell, D. D. Lusterman, & S. H. McDaniel (Eds.), *Integrating family therapy* (pp. 437–455). Washington, DC: American Psychological Association.

Wood, B., Watkins, J., Boyle, J., Nogueira, J., Zimand, E., & Carroll, L. (1989). The psychosomatic family model: An empirical and theoretical analysis. *Family Process, 28,* 399–417.

Wysocki, T., Harris, M., Greco, P., Bubb, J., Danda, C., Harvey, L., et al. (2000). Randomized controlled trial of behavioral therapy for families of adolescents with insulin-dependent diabetes mellitus. *Journal of Pediatric Psychology, 25,* 23–33.

Wysocki, T., Miller, K., Greco, P., Harris, M., Harvey, L., Taylor, A., et al. (1999). Behavior therapy for families of adolescents with diabetes: Effects on directly observed family interactions. *Behavior Therapy, 30,* 507–525.

Young, G. (1973). The treatment of childhood encopresis by conditioned gastro-ileal reflex. *Behavior Research and Therapy, 11,* 499–503.

Zelikovsky, N., Rodrigue, J., Gidycz, C., & Davis, M. (2000). Cognitive behavioral and behavioral interventions help young children cope during voiding cystourethrogram. *Journal of Pediatric Psychology, 25,* 535–543.

Zempsky, W., Schechter, N., Altman, A., & Weisman, S. (2004). The management of pain. In A. Altman (Ed.), *Supportive care of children with cancer: Current therapy and guidelines from the Children's Oncology Group* (3rd ed., pp. 200–220). Baltimore: Johns Hopkins University Press.

Index

activities, pediatric psychology, 9–10
adherence. *See also* family therapy
  asthma, 86, 88–89, 102
  beliefs and culture, 100–101
  challenges to interventions, 99–103
  compliance, 99
  consequences of nonadherence, 86
  cystic fibrosis (CF), 87
  definition, 99
  diabetes, 90, 101–102
  family and, 101–102
  improving, to single components of CF regimen, 143–148
  improving dietary, in practice for CF treatment, 147–148
  interventions to improve, to multiple components of CF regimen, 149–151
  intervention studies published since 2001, 87–89
  Journal of Pediatric Psychology's Empirically Supported Treatments Series, 86–87
  juvenile rheumatoid arthritis (JRA), 87
  limitations of existing language, 99–100
  measurement issues, 100
  parenting style affecting, 102
  school and peer influences, 103
adolescents. *See also* family therapy
  adherence in diabetes, 101–102
  normalizing, rebellion, 90–93
  problem-solving methods, 28–30
adversity–beliefs–consequences (ABC) model, cancer survival 52, 53–54
alarm clock method, tailored, for enuresis, 112
Analgesia Protocol for Procedures in Oncology, systemic intervention, 48
anal sphincter biofeedback, encopresis, 121
anger control, CALMDOWN, 30–31
anxiety, cognitive coping skills, 32–33
asthma
  adherence and family, 86, 102

adherence intervention studies since 2001, 88–89
autogenic training, relaxation, 22
awakenings. *See also* scheduled awakenings

bedtime refusal. *See also* sleep problems
  reviews of treatments, 4, 6
bedwetting. *See* nocturnal enuresis
behavioral family systems therapy (BFST)
  adherence to treatment for cystic fibrosis, 149–150
  diabetes control or adherence, 41
Behavioral Intervention for Change Around Growth and Energy (Be in CHARGE!), cystic fibrosis treatment, 42
behavioral interventions
  encopresis in practice, 122–125
  encopresis studies published since 1998, 121–122
  pediatric psychology, 5
  plus medical intervention for encopresis, 120–125
behavioral techniques
  anger control, 30–31
  autogenic training, 22
  cognitive coping skills training, 32–34
  deepening technique, 26
  diaphragmatic breathing, 23
  imagery-based relaxation, 22, 27
  meditative breathing, 22–23
  preparing child for relaxation procedure, 23–24
  problem-solving methods, 28–30
  progressive muscle relaxation, 23
  recommendations, 34–35
  relaxation training, 21–23
  sample relaxation procedure, 25–28
  urine alarms in combination with, 109–111
  whole-body relaxation, 25–26
beliefs, adherence, 100–101
biofeedback
  clinical issues of encopresis, 126–127